Essentials of

Radiologic
Science

Workbook

Essentials of

Radiologic Science

Workbook

Robert Fosbinder
Starla Mason

 Wolters Kluwer | Lippincott Williams & Wilkins
Health

Philadelphia • Baltimore • New York • London
Buenos Aires • Hong Kong • Sydney • Tokyo

Acquisitions Editor: Pete Sabatini
Product Director: Eric Branger
Product Manager: Amy Millholen
Marketing Manager: Shauna Kelley
Artist: Jonathan Dimes
Compositor: SPi Global
Printer: RR Donnelley – Shenzhen

351 West Camden Street   Two Commerce Square
Baltimore, Maryland 21201   2001 Market Street
                                Philadelphia, Pennsylvania 19103

Printed in China

ISBN-10: 0-7817-7556-6
ISBN-13: 978-0-7817-7556-4

To purchase additional copies of this book, call our customer service department at **(800) 638-3030** or fax orders to **(301) 824-7390**. International customers should call **(301) 714-2324**.

Visit Lippincott Williams & Wilkins on the Internet: http://www.LWW.com. Lippincott Williams & Wilkins customer service representatives are available from 8:30 am to 6:00 pm, EST.

12

1 2 3 4 5 6 7 8 9 10

Dedication

This Workbook is dedicated to my husband, Tom, and my children, Camden and Colin, who grew up with radiography as daily dinner conversation. This Workbook is also dedicated to all of my current and past radiography students for being the guinea pigs for most of these labs—we all learned and experimented together!

Starla Mason

Preface

The *Essentials of Radiologic Science Workbook* is designed to supplement the textbook, *Essentials of Radiologic Science* by Robert Fosbinder and Denise Orth. Each worksheet is directly correlated to a chapter in the textbook and contains Registry-style multiple choice questions, image labeling exercises of selected illustrations in *Essentials of Radiologic Science*, and a crossword puzzle of important terms.

The worksheets can be used as a natural extension of the textbook for outside assignment purposes, and some of the labeling activities can be used to supplement and enhance class activities. Every effort has been made to make the material correlate to the textbook to allow for self-directed student learning, but also challenging enough for test review purposes. The crossword puzzles provide an enjoyable way for students to learn and/or review terms and concepts relevant to each chapter.

The *Workbook* also contains twenty laboratory experiments relevant to the concepts covered in *Essentials of Radiologic Science*, providing students with opportunities to directly apply their learning with hands-on activities. They are arranged in order of the concepts covered

in the textbook and cover basic physics principles in addition to some of the more traditional technique and exposure lab experiments. Each laboratory experiment provides instructions for completing the lab, tables or space for collecting data, and four to seven analysis questions to enhance students' critical thinking skills. Recognizing that digital imaging is now the norm in most radiology departments, five of the experiments are dedicated to CR and DR imaging concepts, and the ability to use computed radiography or direct radiography for collecting data for several of the other labs has also been incorporated.

The *Workbook* has been developed to assist both the educator and student in reinforcing radiologic concepts and to also ensure that the student remains an active participant in the learning process. When used in conjunction with *Essentials of Radiologic Science* and the other ancillaries, such as the videos, animations, PowerPoint slides, test bank, and lesson plans, the *Workbook* is an essential component to complete the teaching-learning cycle.

Starla Mason

User's Guide

This User's Guide introduces you to the helpful features of *Essentials of Radiologic Science Workbook* that enable you to quickly master new concepts and put your new skills into practice.

Workbook features to increase understanding and enhance retention of the material include:

Registry-style multiple choice review questions

Radiation Units, Atoms, and Atomic Structure

1. The Bohr model of the atom consists of a dense _____
   a. positive nucleus surrounded by a diffuse cloud of negative charge
   b. positive nucleus surrounded by electrons in definite shells
   c. negative nucleus surrounded by a diffuse cloud of positive charge
   d. negative nucleus surrounded by protons in definite shells

2. The electron binding energy is
   a. the energy of attraction between electrons in the shells
   b. the energy required to remove the nucleus from an atom
   c. the energy required to remove an electron from the nucleus
   d. the energy required to remove an electron from its orbital shell

3. The atomic number is the number of _____ in the nucleus.
   a. protons
   b. neutrons
   c. protons and electrons
   d. protons and neutrons

4. The nucleus of an atom contains which of the following?
   1. Protons
   2. Neutrons
   3. Electrons
   4. Gamma rays
   a. 1
   b. 1 and 2
   c. 2 and 3
   d. 1, 2, and 3

5. The periodic table of elements lists the elements in order of increasing
   a. atomic number
   b. atomic weight
   c. atomic neutrons
   d. atomic ionization

6. The atomic mass of an element is designated by which letter?
   a. A
   b. M
   c. Z
   d. K

3

38   Part II: Circuits and X-Ray Production

Image Labeling

1. Label the components of the x-ray tube.

2. Identify the anode angles and their respective actual and effective focal spots.

Image labeling exercises

Crossword puzzles

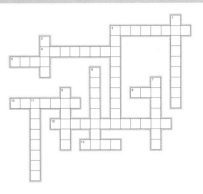

Crossword Puzzle

Across

2. Elements with the same number of protons, but different numbers of neutrons
4. Conventional unit of radiation exposure
5. Emitted from a radioisotope; equivalent to an electron
   ...c mass unit
   ...t of effective dose
   ...o the number of protons in an atom
   ...hemical symbol for this element is Pb

Down

1. SI unit for radioactivity; equal to 1 dps
2. Process of adding or removing electrons from an atom
3. SI unit for absorbed dose
6. Time required for a radioisotope to decay to one half of its initial activity
7. The positively charged center of an atom
8. A nucleon with a positive charge
11. Has an atomic mass of 1/2,000 amu

EXPERIMENT
1

Electric and Magnetic Fields

Name: _____   Date: _____

Electrostatics is the study of stationary or resting electric charges. An electric field exists around all electric charges. An English scientist, Michael Faraday (1791–1867), introduced the concept of using lines of force as an aid in visualizing the magnitude and direction of an electric field. Similarly, the magnetic force per unit pole is called the magnetic field. In this case, the field is mapped out by using the poles of magnets. The purpose of this activity is to allow the student to visualize and map both electric and magnetic fields and compare their similarities and differences.

Objectives:

Upon completion of this lab, the student will be able to:

1. Draw the electric field surrounding both positive and negative charges.
2. Visualize and draw the magnetic field surrounding magnets.
3. Apply the laws of electrostatic and magnetic fields to his or her drawing.
4. Compare and contrast the similarities and differences in electric and magnetic fields and their respective laws of interaction.

Part I: Electrostatic Fields

Draw the electric fields for each charge configuration below, indicating the lines of force, and/or their interactions as applicable. After you have completed your sketches, answer the questions.

a. The electric field of a single point charge
   +

b. The electric field of two like point charges
   +   +

c. The electric field of two unlike point charges
   +   –

Laboratory Experiments relevant to the concepts covered in *Essentials of Radiologic Science* provide students with opportunities to directly apply their learning with hands-on activities.

Reviewers

John H. Clouse, MSR, RT
Deputy Director
Center for Disaster Medicine Preparedness
Department of Emergency Medicine
University of Louisville School of Medicine
Louisville, Kentucky

Anthony E. Gendill, BA, BS, DC
Medical Instructor/Award Winning Faculty Member
Allied Health Department
Institute of Business and Medical Careers
Fort Collins, Colorado

Kelli Haynes, MSRS, RT (R)
Director of Undergraduate Studies/Associate Professor/
Graduate Faculty
Radiologic Sciences
Northwestern State University
Shreveport, Louisiana

Judy Lewis, MEd
Program Director/Instructor
Radiologic Technology
Mississippi Gulf Coast Community College
Gautier, Mississippi

Catherine E. Nobles, RT (R), MEd
Didactic/Clinical Instructor
Radiography Program
Houston Community College System
Houston, Texas

Denise Orth, MS, BS, RT (R) (M)
Assistant Professor
Allied Health
Fort Hays State University
Hays, Kansas

George Pales, PhD, RT (R) (MR) (T)
Radiography Program Director
Health Physics and Clinical Sciences
University of Nevada, Las Vegas
Las Vegas, Nevada

Lisa F. Schmidt, PhD, RT (R) (M)
Program Director
Radiography
Pima Medical Institute
Chula Vista, California

Deena Slockett, MBA
Program Coordinator/Associate Professor
Radiologic Sciences
Florida Hospital College of Health Sciences
Orlando, Florida

Acknowledgments

Special thanks go to Peter Sabatini and Amy Millholen for the opportunity to be a part of this project and for their support and guidance throughout the process of developing the *Workbook*, in addition to all of the ancillaries. A major contributor to this *Workbook* is Jonathan Dimes, who was able to translate my directions and transform various illustrations into student-friendly labeling activities. I would also like to thank the rest of the production staff who have designed the graphics and material together into one professional package.

Many thanks to my family, friends, and colleagues for their support. Thanks also needs to go to my early radiography mentors—your willingness to share your knowledge set me on the path of this most rewarding career. Finally, I am grateful to my husband, Tom. No one could ask for a better supporter or cheerleader.

Starla Mason

Contents

● PART IV: SPECIAL IMAGING TECHNIQUES

● PART V: RADIATION PROTECTION

● PART VI: PATIENT CARE

● LABORATORY EXPERIMENTS

Basic Physics

Radiation Units, Atoms, and Atomic Structure

1. The Bohr model of the atom consists of a dense _____.

   a. positive nucleus surrounded by a diffuse cloud of negative charge
   b. positive nucleus surrounded by electrons in definite shells
   c. negative nucleus surrounded by a diffuse cloud of positive charge
   d. negative nucleus surrounded by protons in definite shells

2. The electron binding energy is

   a. the energy of attraction between electrons in the shells
   b. the energy required to remove the nucleus from an atom
   c. the energy required to remove an electron from the nucleus
   d. the energy required to remove an electron from its orbital shell

3. The atomic number is the number of _____ in the nucleus.

   a. protons
   b. neutrons
   c. protons and electrons
   d. protons and neutrons

4. The nucleus of an atom contains which of the following?

   1. Protons
   2. Neutrons
   3. Electrons
   4. Gamma rays

   a. 1
   b. 1 and 2
   c. 2 and 3
   d. 1, 2, and 3

5. The periodic table of elements lists the elements in order of increasing

   a. atomic number
   b. atomic weight
   c. atomic neutrons
   d. atomic ionization

6. The atomic mass of an element is designated by which letter?

   a. A
   b. M
   c. Z
   d. K

7. Which types of particulate radiation are given off when a radioisotope decays?

   1. Beta
   2. Gamma
   3. Alpha

   a. 1 only
   b. 2 only
   c. 1 and 2
   d. 1 and 3

8. Calculate the total number of electrons present in an atom when there are five orbital shells.

   a. 48
   b. 50
   c. 72
   d. 98

9. Which electron shell has the highest binding energy?

   a. P shell
   b. L shell
   c. K shell
   d. Q shell

10. What is the unit of absorbed dose in the SI system?

    a. Curie
    b. rad
    c. rem
    d. Gray

11. If one electron is taken away from a helium atom, the result is

    a. hydrogen
    b. an isotope
    c. an ion
    d. radioactive

12. The letter designation for the fourth shell out from the nucleus is

    a. D
    b. K
    c. L
    d. N

13. The maximum number of electrons that the P orbital shell can theoretically hold is

    a. 2
    b. 8
    c. 36
    d. 72

14. Sodium, potassium, lithium, and cesium are placed in the same group in the periodic table because they

    a. contain the same number of protons
    b. share similar chemical properties
    c. have identical atomic mass numbers
    d. are all radioactive elements

15. Which of the following radiations would not penetrate the skin?

    a. gamma
    b. beta particles
    c. alpha particles
    d. x-rays

16. Atoms of the same element but different mass numbers are called

    a. isotopes
    b. isotones
    c. isometric
    d. isobaric

17. Radioactivity can be defined as

    a. the ability to do work
    b. potential energy
    c. the quantity of any radionuclide decaying in disintegrations per second
    d. the spontaneous transformation of one element into another

18. How much radioactivity would be left after 6 hours for a sample of technetium-99 if the half-life of this radioisotope is 6 hours?

    a. 100%
    b. 50%
    c. 25%
    d. 12.5%

19. How much radioactivity would be left after 12 hours for a sample of technetium-99 if the half-life of this radioisotope is 6 hours?

    a. 100%
    b. 50%
    c. 25%
    d. 12.5%

20. The general term for the two subatomic particles that occupy the massive, central structure of the atom is

    a. nucleus
    b. nucleon
    c. proton
    d. neutron

21. Radiation that has enough energy to eject electrons from their orbital shells is called _____ radiation.

    a. ergonomic
    b. visible
    c. electromagnetic
    d. ionizing

22. A beta particle is most similar to which particle listed below?

    a. proton
    b. helium nucleus
    c. photon
    d. electron

23. The binding energy of a K-shell electron in a tungsten atom is

    a. 184 keV
    b. 74 keV
    c. 69.6 keV
    d. 37.4 keV

24. Which of the following best describes a proton?

    a. a subatomic particle with a mass of 1 amu and a positive charge
    b. a form of electromagnetic radiation
    c. a subatomic particle with a mass of 1/2,000 amu and a negative charge
    d. an atom with the same number of neutrons and electrons

25. The chemical symbol for the element, barium, is

    a. B
    b. Ba
    c. Be
    d. Bm

26. Which of the following elements has the highest Z number?

    a. hydrogen
    b. aluminum
    c. lead
    d. uranium

27. 100 rems is equal to

    a. 100 rads
    b. 1 Gy
    c. 1 Sv
    d. 1 Ci

28. Which of the following information can be found in each cell of the periodic table?

    1. Atomic number
    2. Atomic weight
    3. Atomic charge

    a. 1 and 2
    b. 1 and 3
    c. 2 and 3
    d. 1, 2, and 3

29. Effective dose is calculated to determine

    a. the amount of radioactivity present in an isotope
    b. the number of ionizations present in air
    c. the relative risk of the dose received by various tissues
    d. the energy of an x-ray photon

30. With regard to the structure of the atom, it is and/or contains

    a. mostly empty space
    b. alpha and beta particles
    c. a nucleus with protons, neutrons, and electrons
    d. large enough to see with the naked eye

Image Labeling

1. Complete the table of radiation units by placing the SI and conventional units and their ratios in their appropriate boxes.

Quantity	SI Unit	Conventional Unit	Ratio of SI to Conventional
Exposure			
Dose			
Effective dose			
Activity			

2. Identify the subatomic particles and electron shells as indicated in the diagram below.

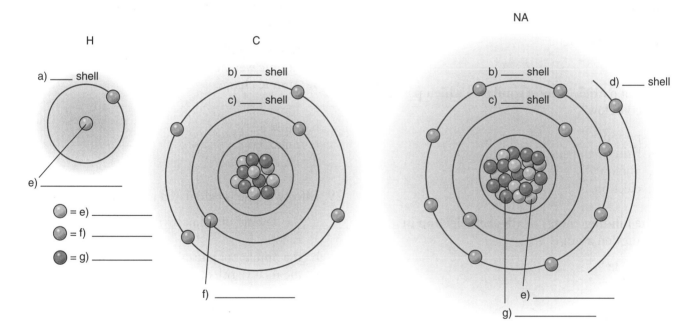

3. Complete the table of atomic mass and charge as indicated.

Particle	Mass in kg	Mass in amu	Charge
Proton	1.6726×10^{-27}		
Neutron	1.6749×10^{-27}		
Electron	9.109×10^{-31}		

4. Label the components of the tungsten atom as indicated.

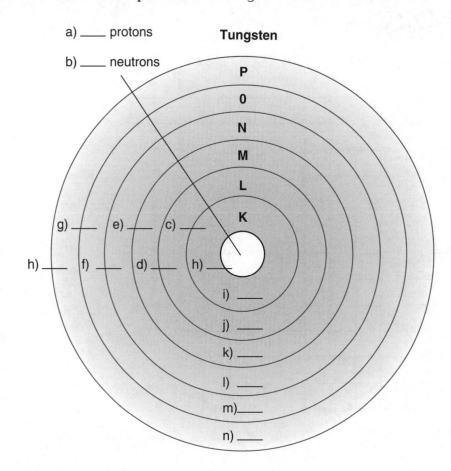

a) ____ protons

b) ____ neutrons

Tungsten

P
O
N
M
L
K

g) ____ e) ____ c) ____

h) ____ f) ____ d) ____ h) ____

i) ____

j) ____

k) ____

l) ____

m)____

n) ____

Crossword Puzzle

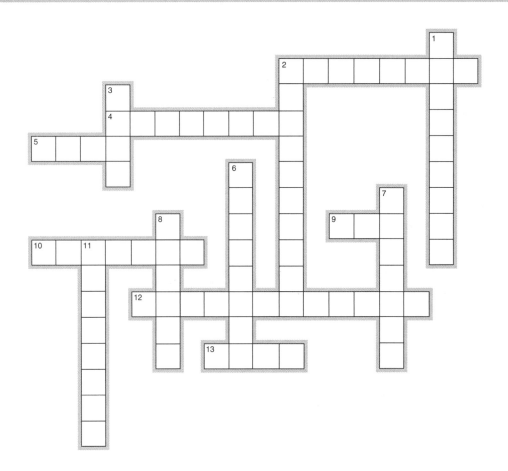

Across

2. Elements with the same number of protons, but different numbers of neutrons
4. Conventional unit of radiation exposure
5. Emitted from a radioisotope; equivalent to an electron
9. Atomic mass unit
10. SI unit of effective dose
12. Equal to the number of protons in an atom
13. The chemical symbol for this element is Pb

Down

1. SI unit for radioactivity; equal to 1 dps
2. Process of adding or removing electrons from an atom
3. SI unit for absorbed dose
6. Time required for a radioisotope to decay to one half of its initial activity
7. The positively charged center of an atom
8. A nucleon with a positive charge
11. Has an atomic mass of 1/2,000 amu

Electromagnetic Radiation, Magnetism, and Electrostatics

1. The unit of electric charge is the

   a. electron
   b. proton
   c. volt
   d. coulomb

2. Which of the following are ways that an object can be electrified (i.e., have charge transferred to it)?

   1. Contact
   2. Rubbing it with a magnet
   3. Induction

   a. 1 and 2
   b. 1 and 3
   c. 2 and 3
   d. 1, 2, and 3

3. The force between two positive charges is

   a. attraction
   b. repulsion
   c. zero

4. The force between a positive and negative charge is

   a. attraction
   b. repulsion
   c. zero

5. The force between two negative charges is

   a. attraction
   b. repulsion
   c. zero

6. The force between two uncharged particles is

   a. attraction
   b. repulsion
   c. zero

7. According to the laws of electrostatics, charge is transferred by the movement of

   a. protons
   b. neutrons
   c. electrons
   d. photons

8. The units of magnetism are the

   a. grass and tesla
   b. gauss and tesly
   c. gruss and tesly
   d. gauss and tesla

9. Which of these materials is not ferromagnetic?

   a. iron
   b. wood
   c. nickel
   d. cobalt

10. **Which of these materials is ferromagnetic?**

    a. wood
    b. glass
    c. iron
    d. plastic

11. **A ferromagnetic material is**

    a. weakly influenced by a magnetic field
    b. strongly influenced by a magnetic field
    c. repelled by a magnetic field
    d. not influenced at all

12. **Two magnets with the same poles facing each other will**

    a. be attracted
    b. be repelled
    c. experience a force times the distance
    d. experience no force

13. **The Earth's magnetic pole under the ice north of Canada is a(n)**

    a. north magnetic pole
    b. south magnetic pole
    c. ice pole
    d. equatorial pole

14. **When a charged particle is put in motion,**

    a. a magnetic field is created
    b. an electric dipole has been ionized
    c. gamma radiation results
    d. it allows positive charges in a conductor to move, also

15. **Which of the following is not a form of electromagnetic radiation?**

    a. microwaves
    b. ultrasound
    c. infrared
    d. x-rays

16. **Electromagnetic radiation travels in packets of energy called**

    a. photons
    b. protons
    c. rays
    d. coulombs

17. **Place the following electromagnetic waves in order of increasing wavelength:**

    1. Visible light   3. Gamma rays
    2. Radio waves   4. Infrared

    a. 3, 1,4,2
    b. 4,1,2,3
    c. 2,4,1,3
    d. 3,4,1,2

18. **Place the following electromagnetic waves order of increasing energy:**

    1. X-rays   3. Visible light
    2. Microwaves   4. Radio

    a. 1, 2, 3, 4
    b. 4, 2, 3, 1
    c. 1, 2, 4, 3
    d. 4, 3, 2, 1

19. **All electromagnetic waves have what characteristic in common?**

    a. they share the same wavelength
    b. they have the same energy
    c. they all have the same frequency
    d. they all travel at c

20. **Light travels at a speed of**

    a. $340 \, \text{mi/s}$
    b. $10,000 \, \text{m/s}$
    c. $3 \times 10^8 \, \text{m/s}$
    d. $2.54 \times 10^{18} \, \text{ft/s}$

21. **Because the speed of light is constant, an increase in frequency results in _____ in wavelength.**

    a. an increase
    b. a decrease
    c. no change

22. **Which of the following statements best describes the relationship between frequency, wavelength, and energy?**

    a. as energy increases, both wavelength and frequency increase
    b. as energy increases, both wavelength and frequency decrease
    c. as energy increases, wavelength increases and frequency decreases
    d. as energy increases, wavelength decreases and frequency increases

23. Using the formula, $c = f\lambda$, calculate the frequency of an x-ray photon that has a wavelength of 2.3×10^{-10} m.

    a. 3×10^8 m/s
    b. 6.9×10^{-2} Hz
    c. 1.3×10^{18} Hz
    d. 7.6×10^{-17} m

24. Using the formula, $c = f\lambda$, calculate the wavelength of an x-ray photon that has a frequency of 3.28×10^{17} Hz.

    a. 1.09×10^9 m
    b. 9.84×10^{25} m
    c. 3×10^8 m/s
    d. 9.15×10^{-10} m

25. The number of wave cycles per second for electromagnetic radiation is the definition for

    a. wavelength
    b. amplitude
    c. frequency
    d. intensity

26. The distance between the same portions of adjacent waves is the

    a. wavelength
    b. amplitude
    c. frequency
    d. intensity

27. The variations between zero and maximum height of the wave is the

    a. wavelength
    b. amplitude
    c. frequency
    d. intensity

28. Hertz is a measure of

    a. the number of cycles per millimeter
    b. the number of cycles per second
    c. energy per centimeter squared
    d. intensity per millimeter

29. One kilohertz is

    a. 1 cycle per second
    b. 1,000 cycles per second
    c. 10,000 cycles per second
    d. 1,000,000 cycles per second

30. One megahertz is

    a. 1 cycle per second
    b. 1,000 cycles per second
    c. 10,000 cycles per second
    d. 1,000,000 cycles per second

31. One hertz is

    a. 1 cycle per second
    b. 1,000 cycles per second
    c. 10,000 cycles per second
    d. 1,000,000 cycles per second

32. Ionizing radiation is radiation that

    a. is continuously emitted from an MRI unit
    b. has enough energy to remove an electron from its orbital shell
    c. is created using ultrasound
    d. causes charge to be transferred through induction

33. If the original exposure rate to a technologist is 8 mR/h at a distance of 4 m, moving to a distance of 2 m results in a new exposure rate of

    a. 2 mR/h
    b. 4 mR/h
    c. 16 mR/h
    d. 32 mR/h

34. Calculate the original intensity given the following factors:

    $I_2 = 270$ mR $d_1 = 40''$ $d_2 = 72''$ $I_1 = \underline{\quad}$

    a. 83 mR
    b. 150 mR
    c. 486 mR
    d. 875 mR

35. Calculate the new distance given the following factors:

    $I_1 = 26$ mR $I_2 = 295$ mR $d_1 = 300$ cm $d_2 = \underline{\quad}$

    a. 30 cm
    b. 89 cm
    c. 600 cm
    d. 1,000 cm

Image Labeling

1. Identify the representative portions of the electromagnetic spectrum identified by the letters below in the order of their increasing energy.

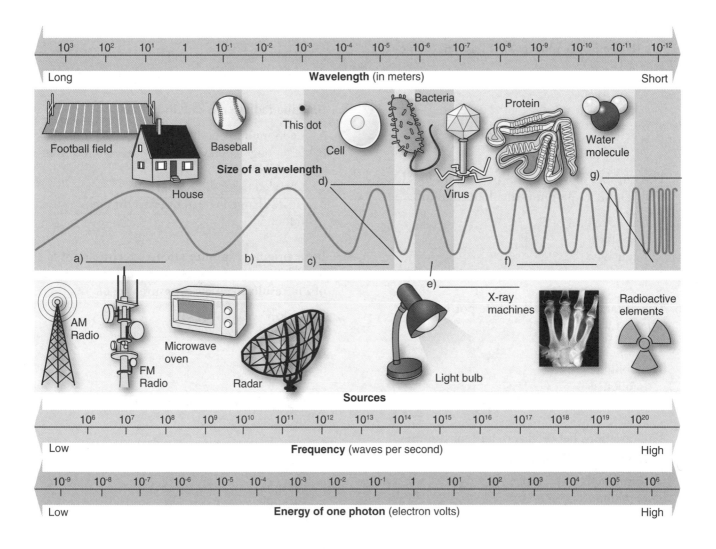

2. Label the identified parts of the wave.

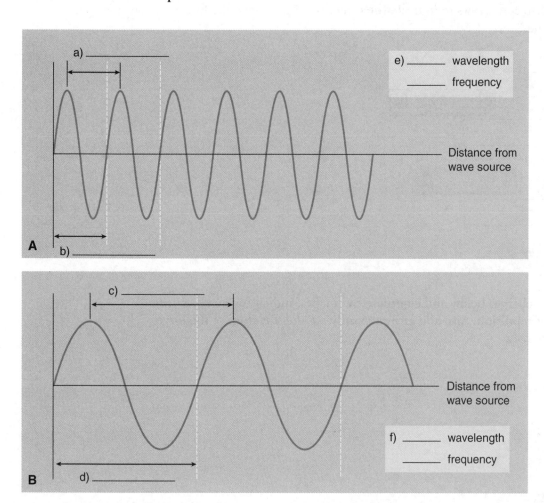

3. Label the identified parts of the wave.

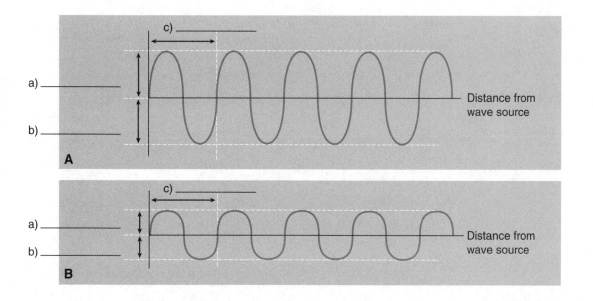

4. Analyze the magnetic poles below and complete each label, indicating whether it attracts or repels. Also add arrows to indicate the direction of the magnetic force between the two poles.

a) _____ poles repel

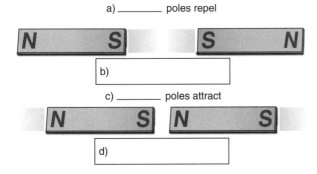

b)

c) _____ poles attract

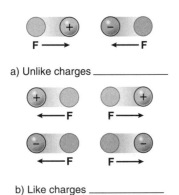

d)

5. Analyze the electric charges below and complete each label, indicating whether it represents attraction or repulsion. Also add arrows to indicate the direction of the force between the two charges.

a) Unlike charges _____

b) Like charges _____

Crossword Puzzle

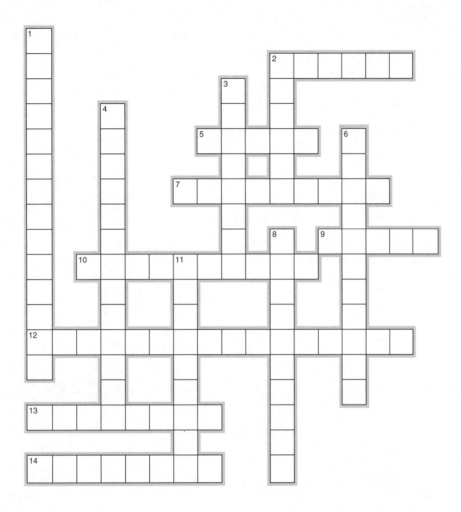

Across

2. The time required for one complete cycle of a wave
5. Unit that measures the frequency of a wave
7. The flux or flow of energy; measured in Wat/cm³
9. The portion of the electromagnetic spectrum with the shortest wavelength
10. The distance between adjacent peaks or adjacent valleys of a wave
12. States that the intensity of the radiation is inversel proportional to the square of the distance (three words)
13. Electrification caused by rubbing two objects together
14. Heat energy

Down

1. Group of atoms with their dipoles lined up in the same direction (two words)
2. A discrete packet of electromagnetic energy
3. The particle that is transferred during electrification
4. Materials that are attracted to a magnet
6. The electromagnetic wave that falls between visible light and x-rays
8. The force exhibited between two unlike charges
11. A natural magnet

Electric Currents and Electricity

1. The four types of electrical materials are

   a. conductors, inflectors, semiconductors, and superconductors
   b. conductors, insulators, semiconductors, and superconductors
   c. convectors, insulators, semiconductors, and supercollectors
   d. conductors, infomers, semicolliders, and superconvectors

2. The unit of electrical potential is the

   a. watt
   b. ampere
   c. volt
   d. ohm

3. What type of material would be the best insulator?

   a. copper
   b. silver
   c. tap water
   d. glass

4. An electronic device that is used to store an electric charge is called a

   a. motor
   b. rectifier
   c. transformer
   d. capacitor

5. A superconductor must be _____ to maintain its superconductivity.

   a. cooled
   b. heated
   c. magnetized
   d. energized

6. Increasing the resistance in a circuit results in a(n)

   a. increase in current
   b. increase in voltage
   c. decrease in current
   d. decrease in voltage

7. Which of the following situations would serve to increase the resistance of a wire?

   a. reducing the temperature
   b. doubling the diameter
   c. doubling the length
   d. reducing the distance

8. The equation, $R = V/I$, is used to express

   a. magnetic flux
   b. Ohm's law
   c. power law
   d. conservation law

9. If a current of 0.5 A flows through a conductor and has a resistance of 6 Ω, the voltage is

    a. 3 A
    b. 12 V
    c. 3 V
    d. 6.5 W

10. The current through a 5 Ω resistor connected to a 220 V outlet is

    a. 220 V
    b. 44 A
    c. 1,100 A
    d. 5 Ω

11. What is the power rating of a lamp that carries 2 A at 120 V?

    a. 120 W
    b. 60 W
    c. 0.167 W
    d. 240 W

12. Voltage can be induced in a wire by

    a. moving a magnet near the wire
    b. placing the south pole of a magnet near the north pole of another magnet
    c. rubbing magnets together
    d. connecting it to a galvanometer

13. According to electromagnetic induction principles, which of the following situations will serve to increase the amount of voltage produced?

    a. increasing the number of loops in the wire
    b. changing the motion of the magnet from 90 degrees to parallel
    c. stopping the motion of the magnet
    d. slowing the motion of the coil

14. An electric motor converts

    a. mechanical energy to electrical energy
    b. electrical energy to mechanical energy
    c. electrical energy to chemical energy
    d. chemical energy to electrical energy

15. The force needed to pass a current of one ampere through a resistance of 1 Ω is the definition for the

    a. volt
    b. work
    c. ampere
    d. watt

16. Amperage is used to define

    a. the direction of flow of electrons through a conductor
    b. the electromotive force impressed on the conductor
    c. the resistance offered by the flow of electricity
    d. a Coulomb of charge passing a given point in one second

17. The core of an electromagnet should be made of

    a. silver
    b. iron
    c. tungsten
    d. copper

18. An excessive amount of electrons at one end of a conductor and a deficiency at the other end is known as

    a. space charge
    b. resistance
    c. potential difference
    d. impedance

19. A coiled helix carrying an electric current is known as a

    a. generator
    b. rectifier
    c. transformer
    d. solenoid

20. Mechanical energy can be converted into electrical energy by a

    a. capacitor
    b. generator
    c. battery
    d. motor

21. A changing magnetic field produces

    a. insulation
    b. sound waves
    c. an electric field
    d. electromagnetic radiation

22. Maximum induction will occur when a conductor cuts a magnetic field at what angle?

    a. 0 degrees
    b. 45 degrees
    c. 90 degrees
    d. 180 degrees

23. A solenoid with an iron core in its center is called a(n)

    a. motor
    b. alternator
    c. generator
    d. electromagnet

24. In a 60-cycle alternating current, how many complete cycles are there every second?

    a. 30
    b. 60
    c. 120
    d. 180

25. What type of motor drives the rotating anode in the x-ray tube?

    a. synchronous
    b. induction
    c. direct current
    d. inductive reactance

26. Electric insulators

    a. store electric charge
    b. permit the movement of electric charge
    c. inhibit the movement of electric charge
    d. change electric charges from positive to negative

27. The unit of electrical power is the

    a. ohm
    b. volt
    c. ampere
    d. watt

28. A simple DC generator is similar to an AC generator except that a DC generator is constructed with

    a. an armature
    b. slip rings
    c. commutator
    d. brushes

29. During the process of mutual induction

    a. electron flow is impeded
    b. current flows in only one direction
    c. current is transferred from one coil to another
    d. a semiconductor becomes magnetized

30. The normal flow of electrons in an x-ray tube is from a _____ cathode to a _____ anode.

    a. negative; positive
    b. positive; negative
    c. cold; hot
    d. magnetic south; magnetic north

Image Labeling

1. Analyze the conductor illustration shown. For lines a and b, indicate which arrow is actual electron flow and which is conventional current flow.

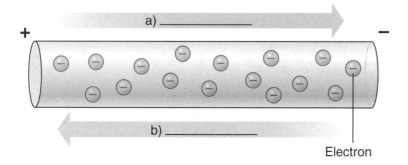

2. Complete the table describing the four types of electrical materials.

Type of Material	Characteristics	Examples
Conductor		
Insulator		
Semiconductor		
Superconductor		

3. Label the electrical components shown.

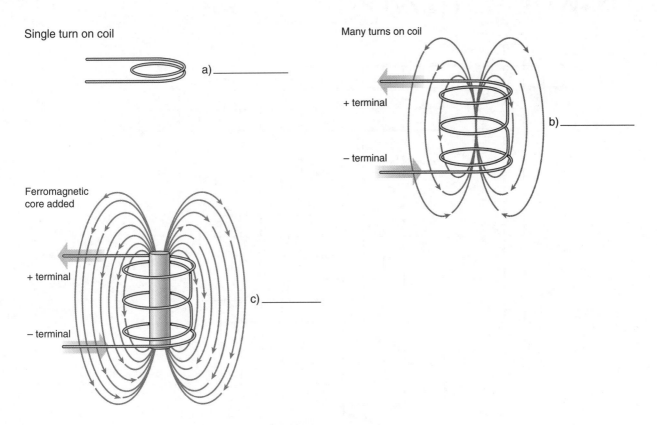

Single turn on coil

a) _____

Many turns on coil

+ terminal

– terminal

b) _____

Ferromagnetic
core added

+ terminal

– terminal

c) _____

4. Label the components of the mutual induction process.

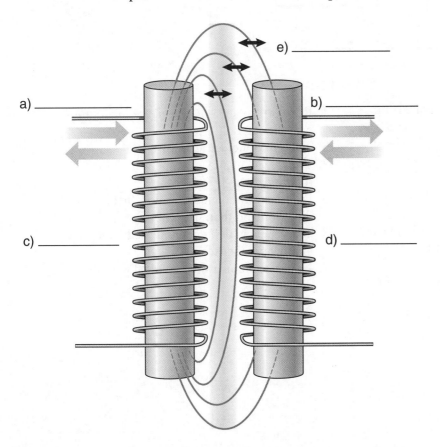

e) _____

a) _____

b) _____

c) _____

d) _____

Crossword Puzzle

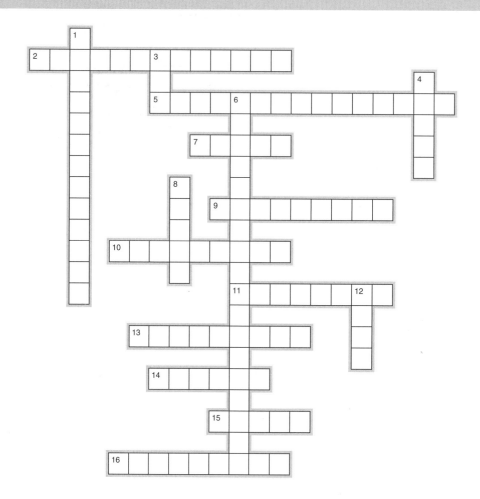

Across

2. A device that contains an iron core in coiled conductor; a mechanism used to produce current
5. Occurs when two coils are placed close to each other; allows current to be transferred from one to the other without touching
7. Electromagnetic device that converts electrical energy into mechanical energy
9. Material where electrons are held tightly in place
10. An electromagnetic device that converts mechanical energy into electrical energy
11. Actual direction of electron flow; from _____ to positive
13. Material that allows electrons to move freely
14. Unit to measure current
15. Used to measure alternating current's frequency; equal to one cycle per second
16. Electrical device used to store charge

Down

1. Rectifiers in an x-ray circuit are made from this type of material
3. The unit for electrical resistance
4. The device in an x-ray tube, which drives a rotating anode
6. Produced when electrons flow first in one direction and then the other
8. The rate at which energy is used; amount of energy used per second
12. Unit used to measure electrical potential difference

PART II

Circuits and X-Ray Production

Transformers, Circuits, and Automatic Exposure Control (AEC)

1. The difference between direct and alternating current is that

    a. direct current flows from positive to negative and alternating current flows from negative to positive
    b. in direct current, electrons flow in one direction only, and in alternating current, they flow first in one direction and then the other
    c. direct current cannot be used by the x-ray tube, so it must first to be converted to alternating current for x-rays to be generated
    d. direct current flows in a magnetic north to south direction and to switch the current flow from south to north, alternating current must be used

2. A transformer with 300 turns on the primary side, input side, and 40,000 turns on the secondary side is a _____ transformer.

    a. step-up
    b. step-down
    c. autotransformer
    d. shell type

3. A transformer with more turns on the secondary windings than the primary windings would be expected to

    a. increase the voltage and decrease the amperage
    b. increase the voltage and increase the amperage
    c. decrease the voltage and decrease the amperage
    d. decrease the voltage and increase the amperage

4. The step-up transformer in an x-ray circuit

    a. has six moving parts
    b. requires DC to induce a current
    c. requires AC for mutual inductance to occur
    d. operates on both DC and AC

5. What effects does a step-down transformer have on current and voltage?

    1. Current increases
    2. Current decreases
    3. Voltage increases
    4. Voltage decreases
    5. Current remains constant
    6. Voltage remains constant

    a. 1 and 6
    b. 3 and 5
    c. 5 and 4
    d. 1 and 4

6. A transformer has 200,000 turns in the primary and 50,000 turns in the secondary side. The turns ratio of this transformer is

   a. 0.25
   b. 250
   c. 4
   d. 150

7. If a transformer has 200 turns in the primary and 600 turns in the secondary side and the input voltage is 110 V, the output voltage for this transformer would be

   a. 3 V
   b. 36.7 V
   c. 220 V
   d. 330 V

8. Which of the following transformer types is designed with an iron bar placed on both the top and bottom of the core to increase the magnetic field strength?

   a. open-core transformer
   b. air-core transformer
   c. closed-core transformer
   d. shell-type transformer

9. The selection of the kVp for an x-ray exposure is made by changing which component of the x-ray circuit?

   a. rheostat
   b. rectifier
   c. cathode
   d. autotransformer

10. Which of the following is not a source of power loss in a transformer?

    a. eddy current losses
    b. rectification losses
    c. hysteresis
    d. I^2R losses

11. A step-down transformer is used in the filament current to change the incoming voltage and current to which of the following ranges?

    a. 5 to 15 V and 3 to 5 A
    b. 100 to 110 V and 60 to 100 A
    c. 110 to 220 V and 110 to 220 A
    d. 50 to 120 kV and 25 to 1200 mA

12. The component in an x-ray circuit that is responsible for varying current is a

    a. rheostat
    b. capacitor
    c. transformer
    d. rectifier

13. When it is necessary to change alternating current to direct current, _____ are placed into the circuit.

    a. rheostats
    b. high voltage transformers
    c. rectifiers
    d. ammeters

In Questions 14 through 24, match the component of the x-ray circuit with its description.

14. _____ Autotransformer
15. _____ Rectifiers
16. _____ Anode
17. _____ kVp meter
18. _____ Glass envelope
19. _____ Step-down transformer
20. _____ Step-up transformer
21. _____ Filament
22. _____ Cathode
23. _____ Rotor
24. _____ mA meter

a. Negative side of the x-ray tube
b. Measures the EMF in the circuit
c. Converts alternating current to direct current
d. Adjusts voltage downward
e. Source of electrons
f. Positive side of the x-ray tube
g. Contains only one coil; serves as kVp selector
h. Converts voltage to the kilovoltage range
i. Serves to rotate the anode
j. Provides a vacuum environment
k. Measures current in the circuit

25. Which of the following circuits and type of rectification requires two to four rectifiers to be in place?

    a. single-phase, half-wave
    b. single-phase, full-wave
    c. three-phase, full-wave, six pulse
    d. three-phase, full-wave, twelve pulse

26. Which type of x-ray circuit would exhibit frequencies in the 500 to 3,000 Hz range?

    a. single-phase, half-wave
    b. single-phase, high frequency
    c. three-phase, six pulse
    d. six-phase, twelve pulse

27. Ripple measures

    a. total tube voltage
    b. variation between maximum and minimum mA
    c. variation between maximum and minimum tube voltage
    d. total mA

28. A three-phase, six pulse x-ray circuit would exhibit approximately how much ripple in its voltage waveform?

    a. 3%
    b. 13%
    c. 1%
    d. 100%

29. The ionization detectors that are employed in most automatic exposure controlled units are located between the _____ and the _____.

    a. tube; collimator
    b. collimator; patient
    c. filter; grid
    d. patient; image receptor

30. If an imaging department that utilizes an automatic exposure controlled (AEC) unit changes the grid or the image receptor speed, what changes must be made for optimum operation of the AEC unit?

    a. all techniques must be doubled
    b. the backup timer must be inactivated
    c. service should be called to have the AEC recalibrated
    d. detector configurations need to be altered for each exam

31. Which of the following circumstances would cause the backup timer to activate during the operation of an AEC unit?

    a. a tabletop exam is being performed with the chest board selected
    b. the rectifiers cease functioning causing insufficient current to the tube
    c. an extremely slender or pediatric patient is being examined and the normal detector configurations are chosen
    d. the technologist has erroneously selected an option to increase the exposure adjustment 30% when it is not necessary

Image Labeling

1. Label each type of transformer shown.

a) _____

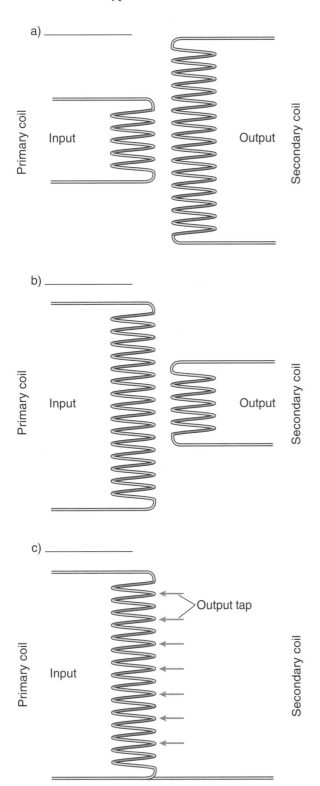

b) _____

c) _____

2. Label the components lettered a through m of the x-ray circuit diagram provided.

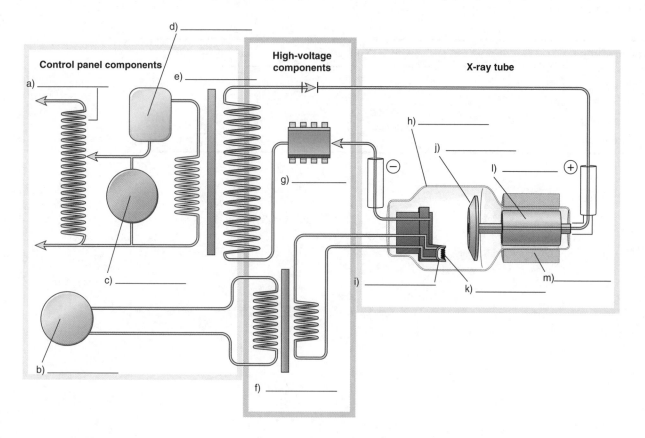

3. Identify each voltage waveform.

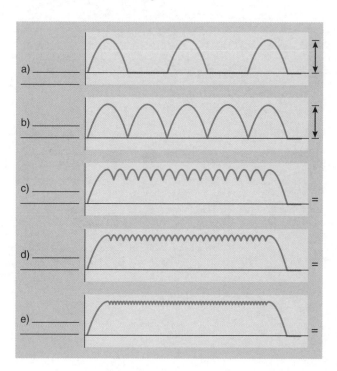

4. For each type of circuit listed, complete the table by identifying its maximum percent voltage and its percentage of ripple.

Type of Circuit	Max % Voltage	Percent Ripple
Single-phase		
Three-phase, six pulse		
Three-phase, twelve pulse		
High-frequency generator		

Crossword Puzzle

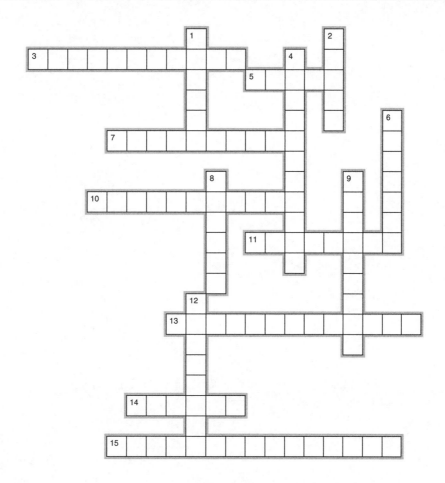

Across

3. Type of current that transformers require to operate
5. Number of detectors most commonly found in an AEC configuration
7. A form of transformer energy loss due to the continuously changing magnetic field
10. Terminates the exposure in an AEC system before tube limits are exceeded
11. Allows resistance to be varied; acts as a milliampere selector for the filament circuit
13. Type of x-ray circuit that exhibits only 1% ripple
14. Type of current produced by rectifiers
15. a device with a single winding used to step up or step down voltage; connected to the kVp selector

Down

1. Amount of variation between the maximum and minimum voltage produced in the circuit
2. Type of transformer constructed with both primary and secondary wires wrapped around its central iron core
4. Electrical device used to increase or decrease voltage
6. In automatic control systems, the detector is placed between the _____ and the image receptor
8. Type of transformer that would have a voltage output greater than the input voltage
9. Device that allows electrons to flow in only one direction; converts AC to DC
12. The step down transformer is responsible for producing the high current needed for this x-ray tube component

X-Ray Tubes

5

1. The heel effect
   a. exists because some x-rays are absorbed by the surface of the anode
   b. is caused by the charge difference between the anode and the cathode
   c. depends on the mA and kVp
   d. is reduced by dual focal spots

2. The principle means of heat transfer from the focal spot to the anode is
   a. conduction
   b. convection
   c. radiation
   d. convention

3. The line focus principle
   a. makes the focal spot appear larger than it really is
   b. makes use of an angled cathode structure
   c. produces x-ray lines
   d. spreads the heat over a larger part of the anode

4. The purpose of the cathode focusing cup is to
   a. alter the filament size
   b. group the electrons for their passage to the anode
   c. regulate anode rotation speed
   d. increase the heat capacity of the tube

If the maximum heat load of a tube in a single-phase circuit is 30,000 HU, which of the exposure series in Questions 5 through 9 is permitted on a cold tube? Answer a for allowed or b for not allowed.

5. _____Five 100 kVp, 300 mA, and 0.25 s followed by one 100 kVp, 100 mA, and 0.1 s exposures

6. _____Five 120 kVp, 200 mA, and 0.2 s exposures

7. _____Five 80 kVp, 400 mA, and 0.2 s exposures

8. _____Six 75 kVp, 350 mA, and 0.2 s exposures

9. _____Five 80 kVp, 350 mA, and 0.2 s exposures

10. A molybdenum shaft is used to connect the anode to the rotor because
    a. it is a less dense metal with a high melting point
    b. it is easily compressed
    c. it has a high inertia
    d. it produces 17.5 keV x-rays

11. Many x-ray tubes have two filaments
    a. because the second filament can be used as a spare when the first one burns out
    b. to provide two focal spots
    c. to allow cooling of the filament by alternating exposures
    d. to improve tube cooling by sharing the heat between two filaments

12. The principle means of heat transfer from the anode to the housing is

    a. conduction
    b. convection
    c. radiation
    d. convention

13. The boost current in a filament

    a. maintains the filament at a standby temperature
    b. is present while the x-ray tube is on
    c. is used to improve the vacuum in the tube
    d. raises the filament to its operating temperature

In Questions 14 through 16, answer a for true or b for false.

14. _____An increase in target angle will increase the heat capacity of the tube.

15. _____An increase in focal spot size will increase the heat capacity of the tube.

16. _____An increase in anode rotation speed will increase the heat capacity of the tube.

The number of heat units for a high frequency exposure of 200 mA, 70 kVp, and 1 s is the maximum allowed. Are the exposures in Questions 17 through 21 also allowed? Answer a for yes or b for no.

17. _____ 100 mA, 70 kVp, and 2 s

18. _____ 400 mA, 60 kVp, and 1 s

19. _____ 100 mA, 110 kVp, and 1 s

20. _____ 350 mA, 70 kVp, and 2 s

21. _____ 200 mA, 80 kVp, and 1 s

22. The transfer of heat by _____ is increased by mounting a fan on the tube housing.

    a. convection
    b. conduction
    c. radiation
    d. convention

The effective focal spot will increase with which of the changes or conditions? In Questions 23 through 25, answer a for true or b for false.

23. _____When changing from 100 to 400 mA

24. _____Increasing the anode angle

25. _____Increasing the anode rotation speed

26. Which of the following does not improve the heat capacity of the tube?

    a. a rotating anode
    b. an increased target angle
    c. larger focal spots
    d. thermionic emission

27. What are the heat units for a high frequency exposure taken at 120 kVp, 300 mA, and 0.6 s?

    a. 22,000
    b. 30,500
    c. 33,000
    d. 45,000

28. The principle means of heat transfer from the tube housing to the room is

    a. conduction
    b. convection
    c. radiation
    d. convention

29. The heel effect is more pronounced

    a. with a smaller SID
    b. with a large focal spot
    c. with a large target angle
    d. with a higher speed anode rotation

30. The effective focal spot is determined by the target angle and the

    a. distance from the anode to cathode
    b. composition of the anode
    c. diameter of the anode
    d. filament size

31. **The disadvantage of a small target angle is**

    a. increased heat distribution and capacity
    b. greater field coverage
    c. a greater anode heel effect
    d. more uniform radiographic density

32. **Thermionic emission is the emission of**

    a. thermons
    b. electrons from a heated cathode
    c. electrons from a heated anode
    d. x-rays from the tube housing

33. **The tube current (mA) is changed by changing the**

    a. filament current
    b. anode voltage
    c. focal spot size
    d. exposure time

34. **To extend x-ray tube life, the technologist should**

    1. **Perform warm-up exposures at the beginning of each day**
    2. **Extend the time that the boost current (prep) button is held down**
    3. **Avoid repeated exposures at or near the tube's capacity**

    a. 1 and 2
    b. 1 and 3
    c. 2 and 3
    d. 1, 2, and 3

35. **Which chart should be consulted to ensure that adequate time has passed before making additional exposures?**

    a. a tube rating chart
    b. an x-ray emission spectrum
    c. an anode cooling curve
    d. a heat unit index

Image Labeling

1. Label the components of the x-ray tube.

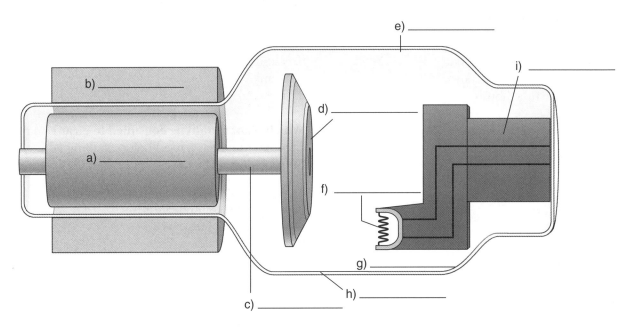

2. Identify the anode angles and their respective actual and effective focal spots.

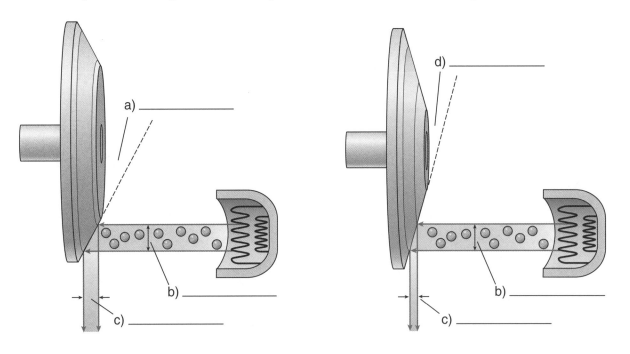

3. Complete letters a through g below, specifying the x-ray intensity range variations caused by the heel effect.

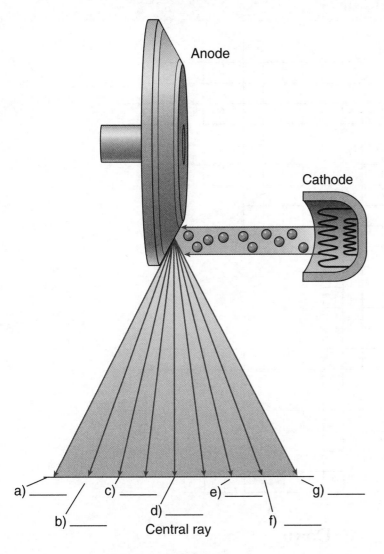

Anode

Cathode

a) _____

b) _____

c) _____

d) _____

Central ray

e) _____

f) _____

g) _____

Approximate intensity (%)

Crossword Puzzle

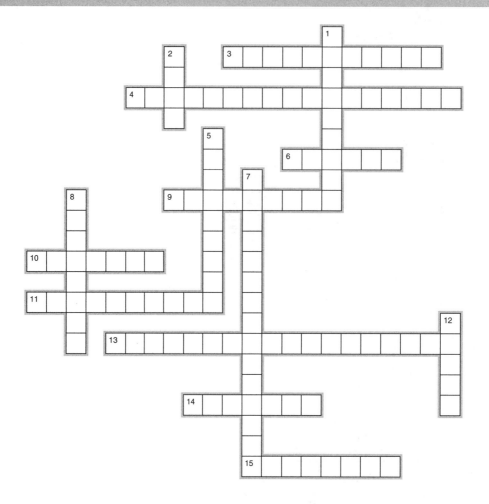

Across

3. Keeps the electron cloud together before they leave the cathode
4. Occurs when no more electrons can be boiled off the filament; limits x-ray tubes to a maximum of 1,000 to 1,200 mA
6. Environment inside the x-ray tube once all air has been removed
9. The product of kVp, mA, and time
10. Type of radiation emitted outside the tube housing; must be less than 100 mR/h at 1 m from the tube
11. Causes uneven distribution of x-ray intensity between the cathode and anode
13. The process of boiling off electrons at the filament
14. The negative electrode of an x-ray tube
15. The anode is constructed of this material due to its high melting point

Down

1. The principle that spreads heat over a greater area of the anode and allows the effective focal spot to be smaller than the actual focal spot
2. Ninety-nine percent of an x-ray tube's output is this form of energy
5. Area where electrons strike the anode
7. Graph that allows radiographers to determine the maximum technical factor combination that is safe for the x-ray tube
8. A coil of wire; source of electrons
12. The positive electrode of an x-ray tube

X-Ray Production

6

1. **Characteristic radiation is produced when**

   a. electrons are stopped at the cathode
   b. a vacancy in an electron orbit is filled
   c. a vacancy in the nucleus is filled
   d. electrons are stopped at the anode

2. **X-ray tube filtration filters out**

   a. low-energy electrons
   b. high-energy electrons
   c. low-energy x-rays
   d. high-energy x-rays

3. **When an incident electron approaches a positively charged nucleus of a tungsten atom,**

   a. the incident electron slows down due to electrostatic attraction
   b. the incident electron penetrates the nucleus
   c. a cascade of electrons from each orbital shell is initiated
   d. a characteristic photon is emitted

4. **As kVp is increased, the production of bremsstrahlung photons**

   a. decreases
   b. increases
   c. is replaced by characteristic interactions
   d. remains the same, but lower energy ranges are observed

5. **If 90 kVp is selected when a tungsten target is used,**

   a. the maximum energy of the projectile electrons and the subsequent x-ray photons will be equal to 30 keV
   b. characteristic photons will be emitted at the 30 and 90 keV
   c. the kinetic energy of the projectile electrons will be equivalent to this energy and the E_{max} of the x-ray beam will be 90 keV
   d. the projectile energy of the incident photons will be 90 keV and the E_{max} of the x-ray beam will be 30 keV

Tungsten has the following binding energies:

Shell	K	L	M	N
Energy KeV	69	11	2	1

6. **Projectile electrons must have an energy of at least _____ keV to produce K characteristic x-rays from tungsten.**

   a. 50
   b. 70
   c. 67
   d. 58

7. More than _____ percent of an x-ray beam is made up of photons produced by the bremsstrahlung process.

    a. 1
    b. 10
    c. 80
    d. 90

8. The cascade process is associated with

    a. molybdenum targets
    b. brems radiation production
    c. characteristic radiation production
    d. filtration effects

9. Bremsstrahlung produces a _____ energy spectrum.

    a. discrete
    b. continuous
    c. kinetic
    d. filtered

10. Which factors affect the characteristic radiation emitted from the x-ray tube?

    a. mA
    b. kVp
    c. filtration
    d. anode material

13. Changing _____ will change the E_{max} of the photons in the x-ray emission spectrum.

    1. mA
    2. kVp
    3. filtration
    4. anode material

    a. 1 only
    b. 2 only
    c. 2 and 3
    d. 2, 3, and 4

14. A technologist can control the quantity of the x-rays striking the patient by adjusting the

    a. mA
    b. kVp
    c. rectification
    d. anode material

15. The maximum kinetic energy of a projectile electron accelerated across an x-ray tube depends on the

    a. atomic number Z of the target
    b. size of the focal spot
    c. kilovoltage
    d. type of rectification

16. Beam quality is primarily determined by

    a. mA
    b. kVp
    c. target angle
    d. focal spot size

17. Beam quantity is primarily determined by

    a. mA
    b. kVp
    c. focal spot size
    d. target angle

18. Which of the following types of radiation cannot be produced at tube potentials of less than 70 keV?

    a. bremsstrahlung
    b. scatter
    c. characteristic
    d. primary

19. The process of removing low-energy photons from the x-ray beam is called

    a. rectification
    b. ionization
    c. electron transition
    d. filtration

20. After electrons strike the anode of an x-ray tube, the majority of the energy is converted to

    a. heat
    b. bremsstrahlung photons
    c. characteristic photons
    d. kinetic

21. Which of the following can be determined from an x-ray emission spectrum?

    1. Photon E_{max}
    2. Photon velocity
    3. Average photon energy

    a. 1 and 2
    b. 1 and 3
    c. 2 and 3
    d. 1, 2, and 3

In Questions 22 through 25, match the x-ray spectrum change with the indicated technique change.

22. _____mA decreased   a. Shifts minimum energy of spectrum to the right

23. _____kVp increased   b. Causes peaks (amplitude) of graph to decrease

24. _____Filtration increased   c. Amplitude, maximum energy, and average energy all increase

25. _____Target Z decreased   d. Characteristic radiation appears in new positions

Use the figure below for Questions 26 through 30.

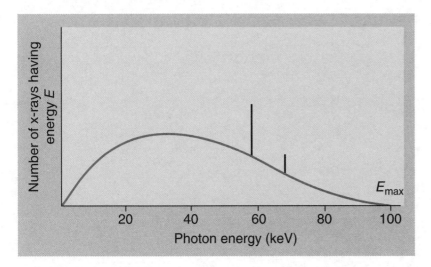

26. The average energy of this beam is approximately _____ keV.

    a. 35
    b. 50
    c. 60
    d. 100

27. The maximum energy of this beam is _____ keV.

    a. 0
    b. 35
    c. 60
    d. 100

28. The energy of the characteristic x-rays is approximately _____keV.

    a. 15
    b. 35
    c. 60
    d. 100

29. The applied voltage that produced this beam is _____.

    a. 20 kVp
    b. 40 kVp
    c. 60 kVp
    d. 100 kVp

30. The heterogeneous wavelengths of this x-ray beam is represented by

    a. the line stretching from 0 to 100 keV
    b. the midpoint of the graph
    c. the spikes shown at approximately 60 and 70 kVp
    d. only the two endpoints of the graph

Image Labeling

1. Evaluate the two diagrams shown and identify each type of x-ray production process being illustrated.

a) _____   b) _____

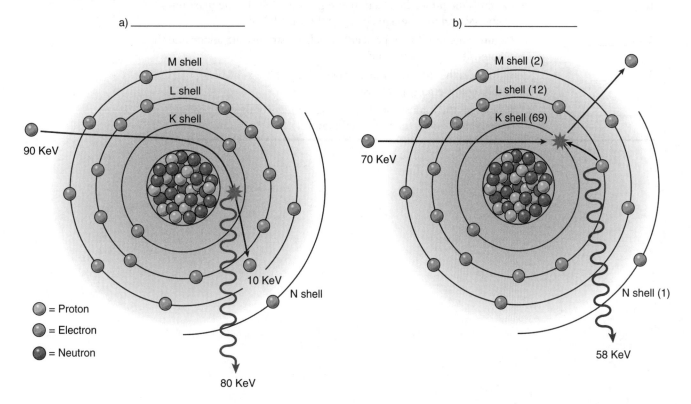

2. Identify the lettered components of the x-ray emission spectra of two different anode materials.

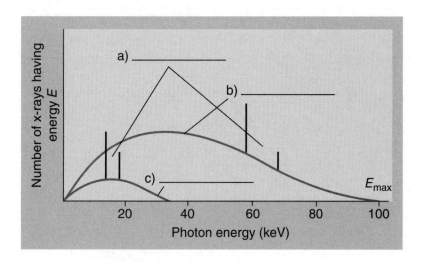

3. **Complete the table by identifying the missing factors that influence the x-ray emission spectrum.**

Other Factors Influencing the x-ray Emission Spectra	Effect(s) on the X-Ray Emission Spectrum
1. _____	Controls the projectile electron energy, the intensity, the maximum energy, and the average energy of the x-ray beam
2. _____	Controls the number of projectile electrons striking the anode and the intensity of the x-ray beam
3. _____	Influences the intensity and average energy of the x-ray beam by eliminating low-energy photons
4. _____	Influences the intensity and the average energy of the x-ray beam by making the x-ray tube more efficient

Crossword Puzzle

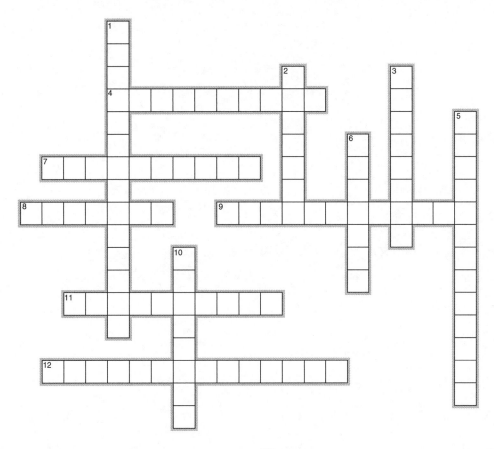

Across

4. Target material used in mammography
7. Eliminates low-energy photons by placing thin sheets of aluminum into the x-ray beam
8. Name for the process of an outer shell electron filling a vacancy left in an inner shell during a characteristic interaction
9. Graph that plots the number of x-ray photons produced as a function of their different energies
11. Brems radiation produces this type of spectrum
12. Type of radiation that results when an L-shell electron fills a K-shell vacancy

Down

1. Type of radiation that constitutes 90% of the x-rays produced
2. Describes the penetrability of the x-ray beam; controlled by the kVp setting
3. Describes the intensity of the x-ray beam; controlled by the mA setting
5. The kVp selected will be equal to this in keV; also called E_{max}
6. Energy of motion; type of energy exhibited by incident electrons
10. Target material with a K-shell binding energy of 69.53 keV

X-Ray Interactions

7

1. _____ is the term used to describe the x-ray beam's reduction in intensity as it traverses through an object.

   a. ionization
   b. attenuation
   c. elimination
   d. transmission

2. **Highly attenuating materials are called**

   a. radiopaque
   b. radiolucent
   c. radioactive
   d. radium

3. **Transmission of radiation occurs when incident photons (are)**

   a. completely absorbed by the nucleus
   b. partially absorbed by outer-shell electrons
   c. deviated in their path by the nuclear field
   d. pass through the patient without interacting at all

4. **What is (are) the product(s) of a photoelectric interaction?**

   a. an electron
   b. an electron and a scattered x-ray
   c. a negative and positive
   d. a photoelectron and characteristic radiation

5. **Which of the following results in total absorption of the primary x-ray photon?**

   a. Compton scattering
   b. coherent scattering
   c. pair production
   d. photoelectric

6. _____is more likely in the case of 40 keV x-rays incident on soft tissue.

   a. coherent scattering
   b. photoelectric interaction
   c. Compton scattering
   d. characteristic radiation

7. **Compton scattering**

   a. involves scattering from the atomic nucleus
   b. involves complete absorption of the incident x-ray
   c. involves a change in direction with no change in energy
   d. involves scattering from outer-shell electrons

8. **Exit radiation is made up of _____ radiation.**

   1. absorbed
   2. scattered
   3. transmitted

   a. 1 and 2
   b. 1 and 3
   c. 2 and 3
   d. 1, 2, and 3

9. The HVL is the amount of material required to reduce the

    a. exit thickness to one-half the intensity
    b. exit intensity to one-half the thickness
    c. exit intensity to one-half the original intensity
    d. original intensity to one-half the exit intensity

10. The HVL in tissue is about

    a. 2 cm
    b. 1 cm
    c. 3 cm
    d. 4 cm

11. The x-ray interaction that involves no loss of energy or ionization is

    a. coherent
    b. Compton
    c. photoelectric
    d. pair production

12. What determines the wavelength of the x-ray?

    a. milliamperage
    b. time
    c. kilovoltage
    d. distance

13. What type of radiation is produced after a Compton interaction?

    a. bremsstrahlung
    b. characteristic
    c. primary
    d. secondary

14. How much initial energy is needed to initiate pair production?

    a. 0.51 MeV
    b. 1.02 MeV
    c. 2.01 MeV
    d. 10 MeV

15. Photoelectric effect occurs when

    a. an x-ray photon causes an electron to vibrate
    b. an inner-shell electron is ejected from its orbit
    c. a positive and negative electron are produced
    d. a nuclear fragment is emitted

16. Which of the following does not involve an attenuation process?

    a. bremsstrahlung
    b. classical scattering
    c. Compton effect
    d. photoelectric

17. The contrast between bone and soft tissue is due primarily to

    a. their similar densities
    b. different abilities to absorb contrast materials
    c. the difference in their atomic numbers
    d. differences in part thickness

18. A radiolucent anatomical structure is one that

    a. easily absorbs x-rays and prevents them from reaching the film
    b. easily transmits x-rays to the film
    c. interacts by the Compton effect
    d. filters out high energy x-rays

19. With increasing kVp and increasing photon energies,

    a. the proportion of Compton interactions increases compared to photoelectric interactions
    b. photoelectric interactions increase overall, while Compton remains constant
    c. the proportion of Compton interactions decreases compared to an increase of photoelectric interactions
    d. as photoelectric interactions decrease, classical scattering becomes the predominant interaction

20. Classical scattering is more likely to occur

    a. in bone and contrast materials
    b. at photon energies of 10 MeV and above
    c. in air-filled structures
    d. when photon energies are 10 keV or less

21. After the nucleus is excited during the photodis-integration process,

    a. a recoil electron is ejected
    b. gamma radiation is detected
    c. positive and negative electrons are produced
    d. a nuclear fragment is emitted

22. During a photoelectric interaction with a calcium atom, the photoelectron is found to have a kinetic energy of 15 keV. The binding energy of the K-shell is 4 keV. Based on this information, what was the energy of the initial photon?

    a. 11 keV
    b. 19 keV
    c. 60 keV
    d. 69 keV

23. An 85 keV incident photon interacts with an M-shell electron of potassium with a binding energy of 35 eV. The recoil electron exhibits a kinetic energy of 29 keV. What is the energy of the scatter photon?

    a. 21 keV
    b. 114 keV
    c. 56 keV
    d. 149 keV

24. Which substance's atoms are the most likely to undergo photoelectric interactions?

    a. barium
    b. soft tissue
    c. fat
    d. air

25. During a Compton interaction, the most energy will be given to the recoil electron when

    a. the deflection angle is 0 degrees
    b. the deflection angle is at right angles to the object
    c. the deflection angle gets closer to 180 degrees
    d. a full 360 degrees is reached

26. An undesirable result of backscatter is

    a. increased patient absorption
    b. increased recoil electron production
    c. increased characteristic photon production
    d. increased image fog

27. Technologist dose is the most likely to increase with the increased incidence of which type of interaction?

    a. pair production
    b. photoelectric
    c. Compton
    d. characteristic

28. Which of the following factors affects half-value layer?

    1. mA
    2. kVp
    3. filtration

    a. 1 and 2
    b. 1 and 3
    c. 2 and 3
    d. 1, 2, and 3

29. Which part of the atom does the incident photon interact with when a pair production interaction is initiated?

    a. an outer shell's positive electron
    b. the nucleus
    c. an inner-shell electron
    d. the nuclear field

30. The interactions with matter of most importance in diagnostic radiology are

    1. Compton
    2. Photoelectric
    3. Classical scattering

    a. 1 and 2
    b. 1 and 3
    c. 2 and 3
    d. 1, 2, and 3

Image Labeling

1. Label the lettered components for the classical scattering interaction shown.

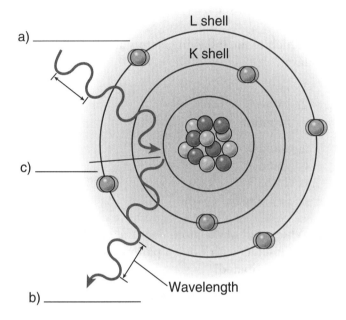

a) _____

c) _____

b) _____

2. Label the steps in the process of the photoelectric interaction in the diagrams provided.

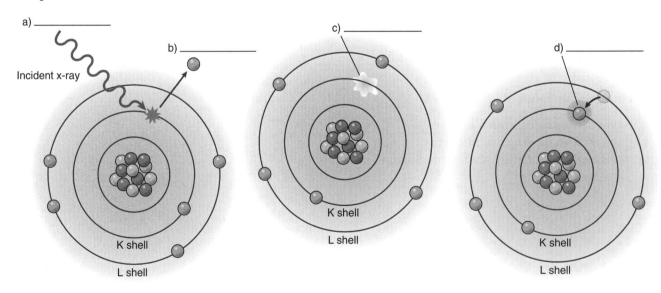

3. Identify the lettered components of the Compton interaction.

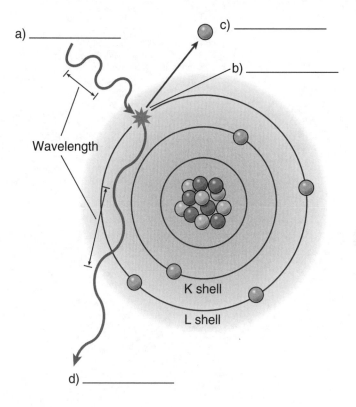

a) _____

c) _____

b) _____

Wavelength

K shell

L shell

d) _____

4. Complete the labels for the pair production interaction.

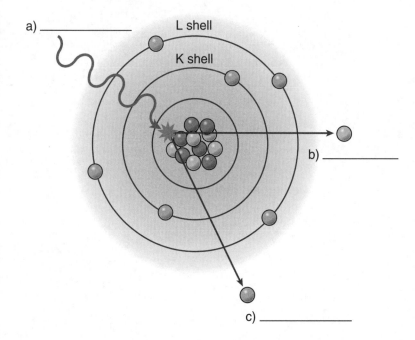

a) _____

L shell

K shell

b) _____

c) _____

5. Complete letters a to c by outlining the steps in a photodisintegration interaction.

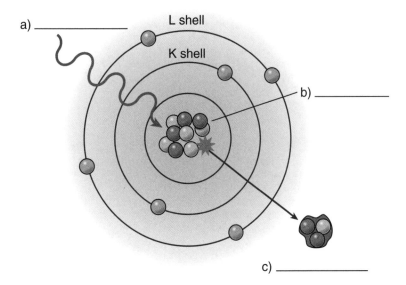

Crossword Puzzle

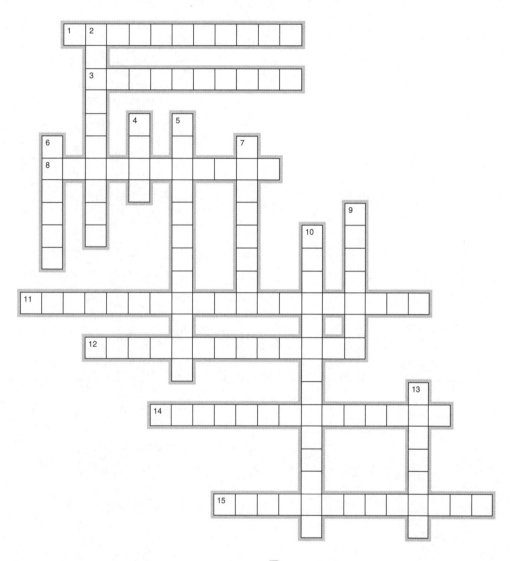

Across

1. Quality used to describe materials with low attenuation values
3. Occurs when a photon is only partially absorbed by tissue
8. Removal of x-rays as they pass through matter due to the complete or partial transfer of photon energy
11. Interaction that occurs in the nucleus of an atom
12. Term used for the electron ejected during a photoelectric interaction
14. Amount of material required to reduce the x-ray beam intensity to one-half its original intensity
15. Interaction characterized by the total absorption of the incident photon

Down

2. Occurs when a photon's energy is completely transferred to the tissue and no longer exists
4. Type of tissue in the body with the highest Z
5. Occurs when radiation passes through a patient without interacting at all
6. Radiopaque contrast medium with a Z of 56
7. Type of scatter produced at energies below 10 keV
9. Interaction that produces the majority of scatter radiation in diagnostic radiology
10. Interaction that results in a positive and negative electron
13. Measured in grams per cubic centimeter

53

PART III

Image Formation

8

Intensifying Screens

1. Spectral matching of the film and screens refers to matching of the

   a. film crystal size to the phosphor crystal size
   b. emulsion thickness to the phosphor thickness
   c. color of the cassette to the film sensitivity
   d. film sensitivity to the color of the light emitted by the phosphor

2. When a medium-speed screen system is substituted for a detail screen,

   a. the patient dose is reduced
   b. spatial resolution is improved
   c. quantum mottle will be increased
   d. patient motion artifacts will decrease

3. Changing from a 200 speed screen to a 50 speed detail screen requires a(n) _____ in mAs.

   a. increase by a factor of 2
   b. increase by a factor of 4
   c. decrease by a factor of 2
   d. decrease by a factor of 4

4. Which of the following films/screen combinations would require the highest mAs in order to achieve the proper exposure?

   a. detail
   b. medium-speed
   c. high-speed

5. Scratches on the screen will appear as _____ artifacts.

   a. negative density
   b. positive density
   c. quantum mottle
   d. fog density

6. Which of the following is not related to the construction of an intensifying screen?

   a. plastic base
   b. phosphor layer
   c. emulsion layer
   d. reflective layer

7. For proper exposure, which type of film should be used with green-emitting rare earth screens?

   a. panchromatic
   b. orthochromatic
   c. duplicating
   d. 105-mm spot

8. Which screen type will result in the poorest spatial resolution?

   a. detail
   b. medium-speed
   c. high-speed

9. Quantum mottle depends on the

   a. K-shell absorption
   b. intensification factor
   c. film/screen contact
   d. number of x-rays interacting in the phosphor

10. Using detail screens with the AEC calibrated for medium-speed screens will result in _____ density.

    a. increased
    b. decreased
    c. unchanged

11. The reflective layer utilizes which of the following materials?

    1. Magnesium oxide
    2. Calcium tungstate
    3. Titanium dioxide

    a. 1 and 2
    b. 2 and 3
    c. 1 and 3
    d. 1, 2, and 3

12. Which of the following are rare-earth phosphor materials?

    1. Calcium tungstate
    2. Gadolinium
    3. Lanthanum
    4. Yttrium

    a. 1, 2, and 3
    b. 2, 3, and 4
    c. 1, 3, and 4
    d. 1, 2, 3, and 4

13. Film/screen contact can be evaluated using a

    a. line pair test
    b. densitometer
    c. wire mesh test
    d. light wavelength measurement

14. If a blue-sensitive film is paired with a green-emitting intensifying screen, which of the following undesirable results is the most likely to occur?

    a. quantum mottle
    b. underexposure
    c. negative density artifacts
    d. increased image fog

15. The purpose of a lead foil liner in the back of a film cassette is to

    a. absorb backscatter radiation
    b. protect the patient
    c. promote photoelectric interactions
    d. reflect light photons back onto the film

16. Which of the following characteristics is desired in screen phosphor materials?

    1. High atomic number
    2. Longer phosphorescence times
    3. High conversion efficiencies

    a. 1 and 2
    b. 1 and 3
    c. 2 and 3
    d. 1, 2, and 3

17. In general, as screen speed increases, density _____ and detail _____.

    a. decreases; decreases
    b. decreases; increases
    c. increases; increases
    d. increases; decreases

18. The primary reason intensifying screens are used is to

    a. reduce patient dose
    b. increase spatial resolution
    c. allow higher mAs techniques
    d. convert light to x-rays

19. Which of the following will have no effect on screen speed?

    a. kVp
    b. mAs
    c. k-edge absorption of the phosphor
    d. phosphor size

20. An imaging department is converting from 200-speed screens to 400-speed screens. A good AP lumbar spine technique using the 200-speed screens is 80 kVp at 32 mAs. What new AP L-spine technique should be used for the 400-speed system in order to maintain density?

    a. 80 kVp at 32 mAs
    b. 80 kVp at 64 mAs
    c. 80 kVp at 16 mAs
    d. 70 kVp at 64 mAs

21. Convert the following technique used on a 500-speed imaging system to a 150-speed imaging system so that density is maintained: 60 kVp 9 mAs.

    a. 60 kVp 4.5 mAs
    b. 60 kVp 18 mAs
    c. 60 kVp 30 mAs
    d. 70 kVp 45 mAs

22. **Which of the following is the most likely to result in quantum mottle?**

    a. a damaged protective coat
    b. poor film-screen contact
    c. large phosphor crystals
    d. low mAs values

23. **The substance with the highest conversion efficiency is the most likely to be**

    a. calcium tungstate
    b. lanthanum
    c. lead
    d. magnesium oxide

24. **The most appropriate measure for an intensifying screen's spatial resolution is (its)**

    a. conversion efficiency
    b. speed
    c. lp/mm
    d. light photon energy

25. **If a cassette "fails" a wire mesh test, what was probably seen on the resulting radiograph?**

    a. numerous negative density artifacts
    b. an area or areas of blur
    c. a clear white grid pattern filling the entire field size
    d. a greenish blue tinge due to spectral mismatching

26. **A film cassette must have which of the following qualities?**

    1. **A radiolucent front**
    2. **Light-proof**
    3. **Even pressure across the film**

    a. 1 and 2
    b. 1 and 3
    c. 2 and 3
    d. 1, 2, and 3

27. **Which of the following screen materials would be the most appropriate to use with orthochromatic film?**

    a. calcium tungstate
    b. titanium dioxide
    c. gadolinium
    d. polyester

28. **If a technologist wishes to improve radiographic detail, she/he should,**

    a. switch to a faster speed screen
    b. use a slower speed screen
    c. use orthochromatic film
    d. make the next exposure using a line pair test pattern

29. **If there is light leak in a cassette, this would be detected due to**

    a. increased image fog
    b. decreased detail or spatial resolution
    c. white, negative density artifacts
    d. mesh-like artifacts

30. **Which of the following is true when comparing rare earth phosphors with calcium tungstate?**

    a. rare earth phosphors possess higher k-edge energies than calcium tungstate
    b. rare earth phosphors emit both blue and green wavelengths of light, while calcium tungstate only emits green wavelengths
    c. rare earth phosphors are able to absorb three to five times more photons than calcium tungstate
    d. rare earth phosphors possess the best absorption properties at the L and M shells, while calcium tungstate relies on K-shell absorption

Image Labeling

1. Complete the steps in the intensifying screen conversion process.

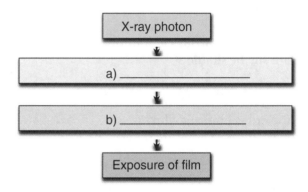

2. Identify the lettered components of an intensifying screen.

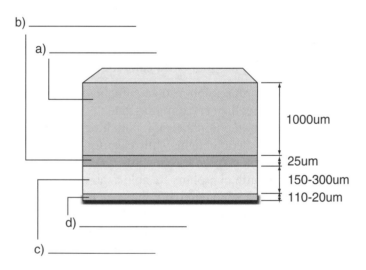

3. Complete the table, indicating the k-edge energy and emitted light color for each phosphor listed.

Phosphor Material	K-edge Energy	Emitted Light Color
Calcium tungstate		
Gadolinium		
Lanthanum		
Yttrium		

Crossword Puzzle

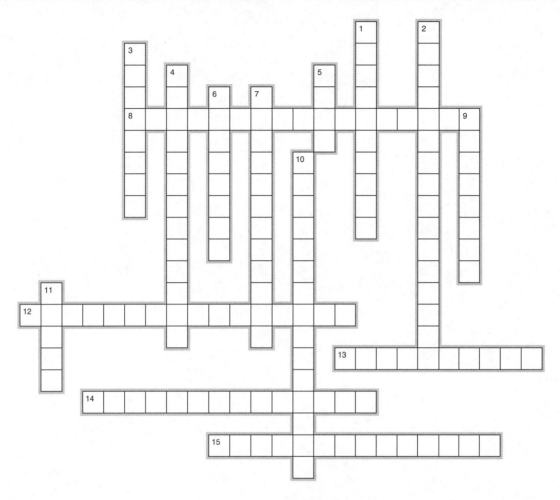

Across

8. Measured in lp/mm
12. Principle that film should be sensitive to the wavelengths of light emitted by the intensifying screen
13. _____ efficiency; measure of a screen's ability to convert x-ray photons to light photons
14. Type of film used with green-emitting rare earth intensifying screens
15. Outer layer of an intensifying screen; covers the phosphor layer

Down

1. Green-emitting rare earth phosphor
2. Blue-emitting phosphor developed by Thomas Edison
3. Crystal that converts x-rays to light
4. Form of image noise; results due to inadequate mAs
5. Layer of the intensifying screen, which is composed of polyester
6. Test that should be conducted if poor film-screen contact is suspected
7. Production of light due to the stimulation of a crystal by x-rays
9. Dust trapped in a cassette results in this type of density artifact
10. Portion of an intensifying screen, which redirects the light back toward the film
11. Numerical measure used to describe screen sensitivity

Film and Processing

1. **A characteristic curve of a film relates**

   a. optical density to the light transmitted through the film
   b. subject contrast to tissue density
   c. optical density to developer temperature
   d. optical density to log relative exposure

2. **The straight-line portion of the characteristic curve of a film can be used to**

   a. determine its base + fog measurement
   b. measure its contrast
   c. find its maximum density
   d. determine the developer temperature

3. **Film base**

   a. provides support for the film emulsion
   b. must have a high opacity
   c. is constituted of gelatin
   d. is chemically reactive

4. **The most common halide used in radiographic film emulsions is/are**

   a. rare earth crystals
   b. gelatin
   c. silver bromide
   d. calcium tungstate

5. **The sensitivity speck is a sensitive region**

   a. in the polyester film base
   b. in the film cassette
   c. on the silver halide crystal
   d. in the developer solution

6. **The latent image is the distribution of**

   a. exposed and unexposed crystals in the undeveloped film
   b. blackened silver halide crystals after development
   c. blackened silver halide crystals in the developer solution
   d. blackened and unexposed silver halide crystals on the undeveloped x-ray film

7. **Optical density**

   a. is always lowest at the shoulder of a characteristic curve
   b. is the logarithm of the ratio of incident to transmitted light
   c. can be measured with a sensitometer
   d. is not affected by light or radiation fog

8. **The diagnostic range of exposures on the straight-line portion of the sensitometric curve falls between**

   a. 0.2 and 3.0
   b. 0.5 and 2.5
   c. 1.0 and 3.0
   d. 2.5 and 5.0

9. The contrast of a film

   a. is measured by evaluating the slope of the straight-line portion on the characteristic curve
   b. is always identical to its speed
   c. is directly proportional to its latitude
   d. is unaffected by changes in processing conditions

10. A high contrast film has a _____ latitude.

    a. wide
    b. narrow
    c. long
    d. low

11. The optical density of a film is measured with a

    a. sensitometer
    b. densitometer
    c. penetrometer
    d. photometer

12. A characteristic curve optical density measurement of 0.3 would most likely be found at the

    a. toe
    b. straight-line portion
    c. shoulder
    d. D_{max}

13. The shoulder of the characteristic curve represents

    a. a film's base + fog measurement
    b. the area of highest film resolution
    c. a film's latitude of exposure
    d. the maximum densities achievable

14. The device that is used to consistently produce a series of density steps progressing from clear to black best describes the

    a. densitometer
    b. thermometer
    c. sensitometer
    d. optimeter

For Questions 15 through 20, indicate whether the property is described by and/or can be evaluated by the characteristic curve. Answer a for true or b for false.

15. _____ Resolution

16. _____ Contrast

17. _____ Base + fog level

18. _____ Latitude

19. _____ Speed

20. _____ Focal spot size

21. A high speed film is one that

    a. requires a high kVp to produce a given exposure
    b. requires a very short development time
    c. requires a relatively low exposure to produce a given density
    d. requires a relatively high exposure to produce a given density

22. A 600-speed system is in general use in your department, but on a particular exam, you switch to a 200-speed system. To maintain density, you will have to

    a. increase technique by three times
    b. increase technique by 1/3
    c. increase technique by 400 times
    d. decrease technique by 1/3

23. Your current technique of 1.5 mAs at 56 kVp is used for a hand utilizing a system speed of 400. A suspicious area on a hand requires a better film, so you switch to a system with a speed of 150. What new technique is required to maintain the original density?

    a. 0.6 mAs
    b. 6.0 mAs
    c. 4.0 mAs
    d. 40 mAs

24. Which of the following would enhance resolution the MOST?

    a. using a film with larger silver halide crystals
    b. using slower speed film
    c. using a film with a thicker emulsion
    d. using a safelight filter

25. The purpose of processing and development is to

    a. create the latent image
    b. enhance radiographic base + fog
    c. minimize artifact formation
    d. make the latent image visible

26. The reducing agents of the developer control the overall blackness of the radiographic image. Of the two agents used, _____ produces the highest density areas and _____ produces the subtler shades of gray.

    a. hydroquinone; phenidone
    b. silver halide; silver sulfide
    c. hypo; phenidone
    d. acids; bases

27. Solution replenishment that occurs in an automatic processor is controlled by the activation of a

    a. master roller
    b. microswitch
    c. circulation pump
    d. guideshoe

28. Total processing time is controlled by which automatic processor system?

    a. thermostat
    b. transport
    c. recirculation
    d. replenishment

29. A radiograph having a density of 1.0 will transmit what percentage of illuminator light?

    a. 1%
    b. 10%
    c. 100%
    d. 1,000%

30. The developer temperature in most 90-second automatic processors is in the range of

    a. 68°F to 72°F (23°C to 25°C)
    b. 80°F (28°C ± 5°C)
    c. 92°F to 95°F (28°C ± 5°C)
    d. 110°F to 120°F (43°C to 50°C)

Image Labeling

1. Label each layer of the double-emulsion film shown.

a) _____

b) _____

c) _____

d) _____

e) _____

f) _____

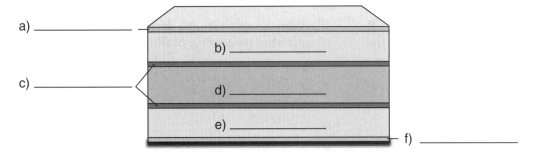

2. Complete the table by demonstrating the relationships of crystal size and emulsion thickness to film speed and resolution.

Relationship of Crystal Size and Emulsion to Film Factors

	Crystal Size		Emulsion Layer	
	Small	Large	Thin	Thick
Speed				
Resolution				

3. Label the parts of the characteristic curve.

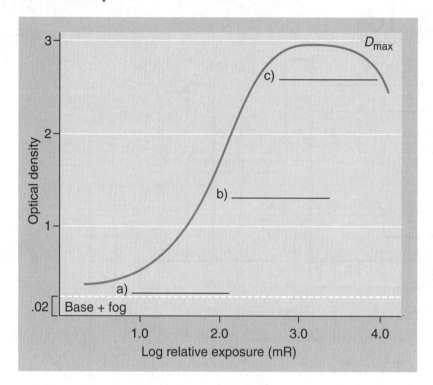

4. Label the processor components.

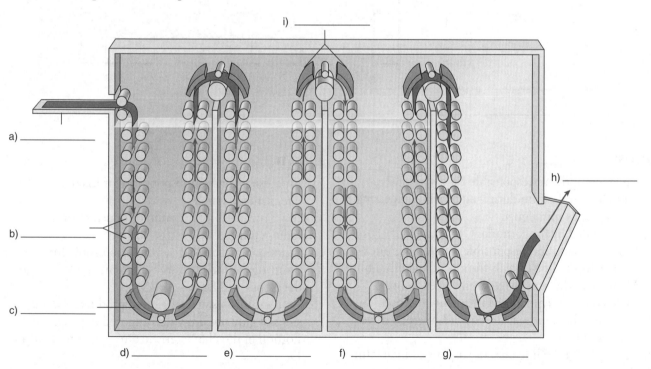

Crossword Puzzle

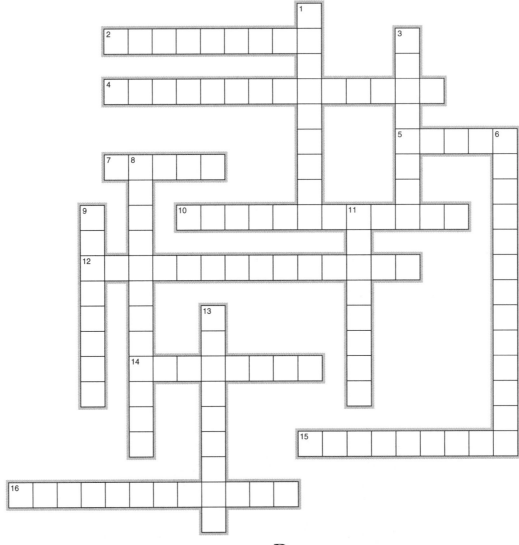

Across

2. Metal component responsible for causing scratches on the film during automatic processing if it becomes misaligned
4. Represented by the formula: OD = log(Io/It)
5. Processing solution responsible for clearing unexposed silver halide crystals from a radiographic film
7. Measure of the sensitivity of film to exposure
10. Most common type of silver recovery method
12. Type of radiographic film sensitive to green wavelengths of light
14. Made of silver halide crystals suspended in gelatin
15. Processing systems in control of the time that the film is in the solutions
16. Measurement of a film's response to processing and exposure conditions

Down

1. Processing solution responsible for making the latent image visible
3. Any unwanted information or densities on a radiograph
6. Automatic processing system responsible for ensuring fresh chemistry is regularly added to the developer and fixer
8. An aluminum step wedge that produces varying steps of gray on film when exposed to x-rays
9. Portion of the characteristic curve used to measure D_{max}
11. Range of exposures that produce acceptable densities in the diagnostic range
13. Material used for the base of radiographic film

10

Density and Contrast

1. Radiographic contrast consists of a combination of

   a. subject contrast and scattering
   b. subject contrast and film contrast
   c. film contrast and grid contrast
   d. density and mAs

2. Subject contrast depends on

   a. tissue thickness
   b. tissue density
   c. tissue atomic number
   d. all of the above

3. Thicker body parts result in greater

   a. transmission
   b. bremsstrahlung
   c. attenuation
   d. tissue density

4. Materials with higher atomic numbers have lower

   a. transmission
   b. bremsstrahlung
   c. attenuation
   d. tissue density

5. Higher energy x-ray beams have lower _____ than x-ray beams with lower energy.

   a. transmission
   b. bremsstrahlung
   c. attenuation
   d. tissue density

6. Iodine and barium are used as contrast agents because they

   a. are liquids
   b. possess higher atomic numbers
   c. have high melting points
   d. are pure elements

7. Long-scale contrast radiographs are obtained using

   a. increased mAs
   b. decreased mAs
   c. increased kVp
   d. decreased kVp

8. The most critical factor in obtaining diagnostic quality images using an automatic exposure control (AEC) circuit is the use of accurate

   a. positioning/centering
   b. focal spot size
   c. side markers
   d. backup time

9. The primary factor that controls density is

   a. kVp
   b. mAs
   c. grids
   d. SID

10. The primary factor that controls image contrast is the

    a. kVp
    b. mAs
    c. SID
    d. focal spot size

11. When utilizing the AEC, changing the mA from 100 to 300 will result in

    a. more density
    b. less contrast
    c. a shorter exposure time
    d. less distortion

12. A radiograph has been determined to have high contrast. This means that the density differences between structures are

    a. relatively small
    b. exactly equal
    c. large
    d. >0.5 on a densitometer reading

13. Scatter and radiation fog have what effect on radiographic quality?

    a. reduce penumbra of the image
    b. create penumbra in the image
    c. decrease the contrast of the image
    d. increase the contrast of the image

14. In order to maintain density, when one increases kVp from 70 to 80, one must

    a. increase mAs by two times
    b. decrease mAs to 1/4 the original
    c. increase mAs by four times
    d. decrease mAs to 1/2 the original

15. Which of the following anatomic structures would exhibit the highest subject contrast?

    a. kidney
    b. heart
    c. wrist
    d. lungs

16. The minimum percent change in mAs required to see a noticeable change in film density is about

    a. 50%
    b. 30%
    c. 0%
    d. 20%

17. The purpose of the backup timer in an AEC system is to

    a. increase the exposure time
    b. allow the ion chambers enough time to respond to the remnant radiation
    c. provide the technologist with a mechanism to verify the actual mAs of the exposure
    d. prevent excessive exposure by shutting the exposure off in case of the AEC's timer switch failure

18. If the original technique used was 60 kVp at 25 mAs, which new technique will result in a film density two times darker?

    a. 64 kVp at 25 mAs
    b. 60 kVp at 50 mAs
    c. 60 kVp at 33 mAs
    d. 60 kVp at 75 mAs

19. Which of the following increases as collimation increases?

    a. density
    b. scatter production
    c. fog
    d. contrast

20. If the SID is increased from 40 to 60 in and the original mAs used is 20 mAs, what new mAs is needed to maintain density?

    a. 10 mAs
    b. 26 mAs
    c. 40 mAs
    d. 80 mAs

21. The use of beam-restricting devices results in a smaller area of exposure on the finished radiograph. This will, in turn, decrease

    a. resolution
    b. density
    c. quantum mottle
    d. contrast

22. In general, as image receptor speed increases,

    a. density increases
    b. contrast decreases
    c. fog increases
    d. resolution increases

23. **In order to increase contrast, the technologist should**

    a. increase mAs
    b. decrease kVp
    c. increase SID
    d. decrease grid ratio

24. **If the anatomy to be imaged is deemed to have low subject contrast, the resulting radiograph will have**

    a. low radiographic contrast
    b. increased radiographic contrast
    c. a short scale of contrast
    d. high-density differences between anatomic areas

25. **Which of the following factors have no effect on contrast?**

    a. focal spot size
    b. kVp
    c. grid ratio
    d. beam restriction

26. **Which of the following occurs when a technologist increases the technique from 200 to 400 mA?**

    a. the x-ray photons become more penetrating and increase density
    b. fewer photons reach the image receptor because kVp is automatically decreased by the x-ray circuit
    c. more x-rays photons are produced, increasing density
    d. lower energy photons are filtered out, making the beam more energetic

27. **Radiopacity will be greatest in which type of material listed below?**

    a. fat
    b. barium
    c. soft tissue
    d. bone

28. **Which of the following statements is true with regard to differential absorption?**

    a. structures with high atomic numbers are more likely to attenuate x-ray photons
    b. differential absorption is similar for all body structures; it is the photon energy that ultimately determines transmission
    c. iodine is a radiolucent contrast agent, while barium is a radiopaque contrast agent
    d. the 15% rule was formulated because four centimeters of human tissue will always absorb nearly 100% of the photons produced

29. **While performing an abdomen examination in the erect position using an AEC unit, you use 72 inches rather than 40 inches SID. The density of this radiograph will be**

    a. unacceptably light
    b. unacceptably dark
    c. acceptable
    d. mottled

30. **After performing two erect views of the shoulder using an AEC, you place the image receptor on the tabletop for the axillary view with no other changes to the control panel. After positioning the patient for the axillary, what is likely to occur?**

    a. no exposure to the image receptor and the backup timer alarm will go off
    b. overexposure to the image receptor and the backup timer alarm will go off
    c. the exposure will be acceptable because the AEC detectors will automatically adjust the time needed
    d. overexposure because the image receptor is on the tabletop and the AEC detector is only used for exposures using the Bucky

Image Labeling

1. Label the amount of density that will result based on the percentage of light transmitted.

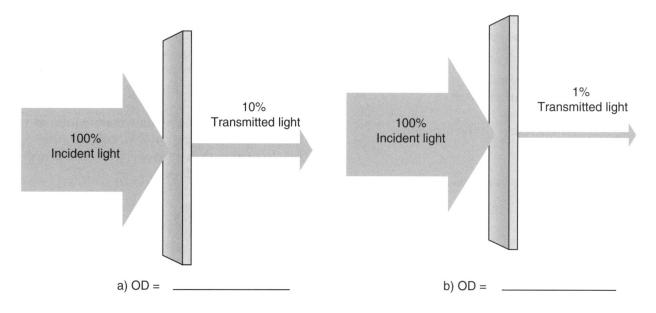

a) OD = _____   b) OD = _____

2. Identify the type of kVp, wavelength, and contrast produced demonstrated in the diagram.

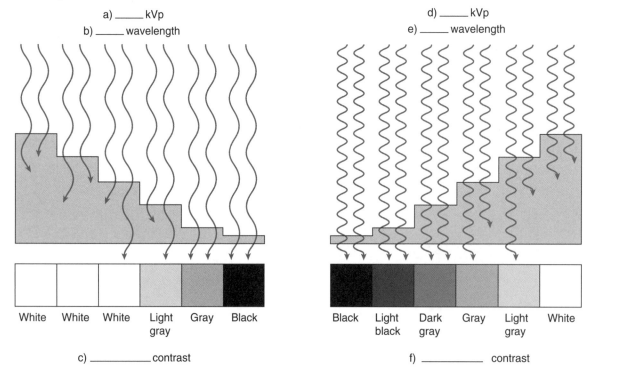

3. Complete the table by filling in the missing terms used to describe contrast.

Terms Used To Describe Contrast

Low Contrast	High Contrast

Crossword Puzzle

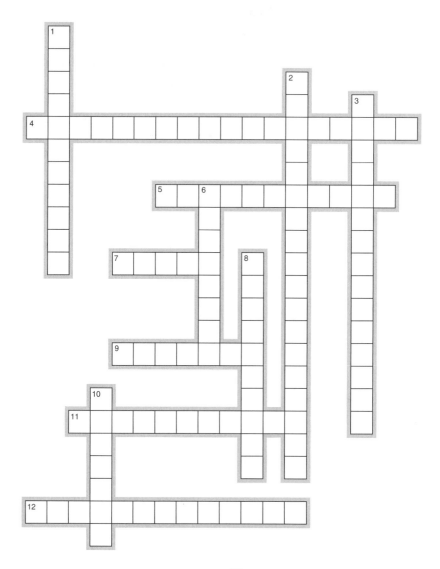

Across

4. Used to calculate the amount of change in kVp needed to double the radiographic density
5. Control on an AEC unit that prevents x-ray tube failure; terminates an x-ray exposure that is too long
7. A high-contrast image produces this type of contrast scale
9. Caused by Compton radiation; reduces image contrast
11. Increasing kVp causes this x-ray beam characteristic to increase, also
12. Barium and iodine are examples

Down

1. Term for beam restriction
2. Formula used to calculate the new mAs when SID is changed
3. Arises from differences in exit radiation from different areas of the body
6. Difference in density between two areas on the image
8. Acts to absorb weaker photons in order to produce a more energetic beam
10. The degree of blackening of the x-ray image

Image Formation

In Questions 1 through 3, match the technical changes with the effect produced on the image (not all answers may be used).

1. _____ Increased kVp

2. _____ Decreased kVp

3. _____ larger focal spot

a. greater unsharpness
b. less contrast, longer scale of contrast
c. lower fog
d. shorter contrast scale, greater contrast

4. Which of the following would improve radiographic quality if patient motion was a problem?

   a. 0.6 mm focal spot, 100 mA, and 0.25 seconds
   b. 0.6 mm focal spot, 200 mA, and 0.125 seconds
   c. 0.6 mm focal spot, 300 mA, and 0.083 seconds
   d. 1.2 mm focal spot, 500 mA, and 0.050 seconds

5. An exposure of 85 kVp and 200 mAs produces a correct density but too much contrast. What mAs should be used to maintain density if the kVp is raised to 100 kVp?

   a. 50
   b. 100
   c. 200
   d. 400

6. If the distance from the source is increased by a factor of 2, the mAs must be _____ to maintain the same density.

   a. increased by a factor of 2
   b. decreased by a factor of 2
   c. increased by a factor of 4
   d. decreased by a factor of 4

7. If the distance from the source is decreased by a factor of 2, the mAs must be _____ to maintain the same image density.

   a. increased by a factor of 2
   b. decreased by a factor of 2
   c. increased by a factor of 4
   d. decreased by a factor of 4

8. The factor that alters image unsharpness is

   a. mAs
   b. kVp
   c. anode material
   d. focal spot size

9. Which of the following has/have no effect on sharpness of detail?

   a. penumbra
   b. motion
   c. density
   d. lp/mm

10. Which of the following techniques would produce the same density as 500 mA at 0.03 seconds?

    a. 300 mA at 0.05 seconds
    b. 100 mA at 0.015 seconds
    c. 200 mA at 0.10 seconds
    d. 250 mA at 0.6 seconds

11. The greater the number of photons (intensity) that reach the image receptor, the

    a. greater the image penumbra
    b. greater the contrast
    c. greater the density
    d. lower the contrast

12. The factor that alters x-ray beam quality is

    a. mAs
    b. kVp
    c. distance
    d. focal spot size

13. An exposure of 40 inches SID, 200 mA, 2 seconds, and 80 kVp is changed to 40 inches SID, 100 mA, and 2 seconds. What kVp should be chosen to produce the same image?

    a. 70 kVp
    b. 80 kVp
    c. 92 kVp
    d. 100 kVp

14. A variation from the true shape of the part being radiographed is defined as

    a. misrepresentation
    b. facsimile
    c. magnification
    d. distortion

15. The following factors could result in significant elongation of an image EXCEPT

    a. shape of the object
    b. tube angulation
    c. tube-grid alignment
    d. tube-part alignment

16. If the central ray is not placed so that it is directed through the center of the anatomy, the radiographic quality most affected will be

    a. density
    b. contrast
    c. detail
    d. distortion

17. An increase in the source-to-image receptor distance will

    a. increase penumbra
    b. increase blur
    c. decrease penumbra
    d. not change penumbra

18. Which of the following would have the most effect on magnification of the image on a finished radiograph?

    a. object-to-image-receptor distance
    b. motion
    c. focal spot size
    d. system speed

19. To calculate the magnification factor,

    a. divide the SID by the OID
    b. divide the object size by the image size
    c. divide the SID by the SOD
    d. divide the OID by the SID

20. An image of the sacrum measures 17 cm long on the film. The radiograph was taken under the following conditions: SID = 100 cm and OID = 8.4 cm. Calculate and select the correct magnification factor.

    a. 1.33
    b. 1.09
    c. 11.9
    d. 1.2

21. The larger the tomographic angle, the

    a. thicker the cut or object plane
    b. thinner the cut or object plane
    c. faster the cut
    d. larger the body part

22. The advantage of tomography is improved

    a. density
    b. ability to see superimposed structures
    c. detail
    d. patient exposure

23. The location of the object plane is determined by the

    a. focal spot size
    b. tomographic angle
    c. SID
    d. fulcrum location

24. A radiograph of the sella turcica was performed using an SID of 40 inches. The sella turcica has a 10 inches OID. What is the magnification factor of the sella turcica?

    a. 0.25
    b. 0.75
    c. 1.33
    d. 4.0

25. At 60 inches the x-ray intensity is 90 mR. What is the intensity at 36 inches?

    a. 36 mR
    b. 18 mR
    c. 250 mR
    d. 360 mR

26. A UGI image is blurred. Based on the type of exam being conducted, to increase sharpness of detail, the technologist could

    a. decrease exposure time
    b. use a single screen cassette
    c. decrease kVp and mAs
    d. decrease SID

27. Which of the following combinations of factors will provide the greatest detail?

    a. Short SID, short OID, and small FSS
    b. Long SID, short OID, and small FSS
    c. Long SID, long OID, and large FSS
    d. Short SID, long OID, and large FSS

28. Size distortion will be affected by all of the following EXCEPT

    a. SID
    b. SOD
    c. OID
    d. FSS

29. Bone mineral densitometry is a special imaging technique used to

    a. align anatomical structures
    b. produce thinner sections of anatomy
    c. eliminate motion blur
    d. measure the amount of trabeculae present

30. During linear tomography, which of the following motions are synchronized?

    a. x-ray tube and image receptor
    b. x-ray tube anode and cathode
    c. image receptor and the object
    d. image receptor and the Bucky

Image Labeling

1. Identify the type of distance indicated in the diagram.

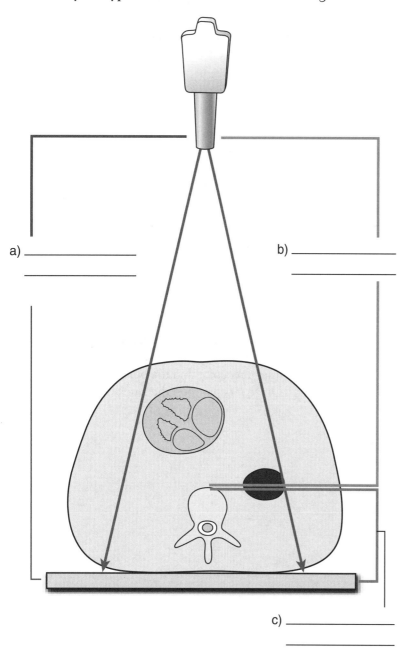

a) _____

_____

b) _____

_____

c) _____

_____

2. Indicate whether the SID and OID are large or small based on the diagram.

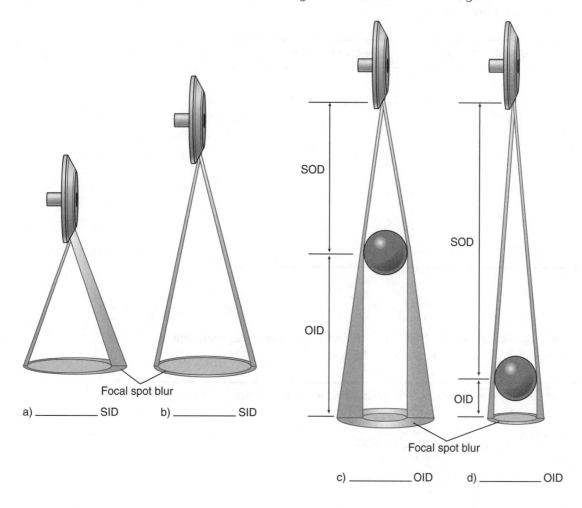

a) _____ SID   b) _____ SID

c) _____ OID   d) _____ OID

3. Identify whether the anatomy is elongated or foreshortened.

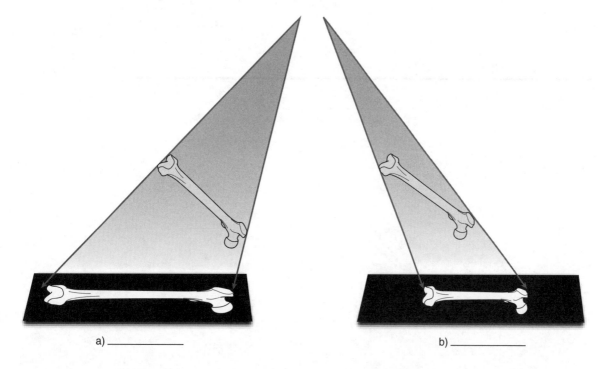

a) _____   b) _____

4. Complete the table by indicating whether the factor will increase or decrease density and contrast or will remain unchanged.

Factor	Density Change	Contrast Change
mA increase		
mA decrease		
Time increase		
Time decrease		
kVp increase		
kVp decrease		
SID increase		
SID decrease		
Focal spot increase		
Focal spot decrease		

5. Complete the table by indicating whether the factor will increase or decrease the image qualities shown or if they will remain unchanged.

Factor	Patient Dose	Magnification	Focal Spot Blur	Motion Blur	Film Density
Film speed					
Screen speed					
Grid ratio					
Patient thickness					
Focal spot size					
SID					
OID					
mAs					
Exposure time					
kVp					

Crossword Puzzle

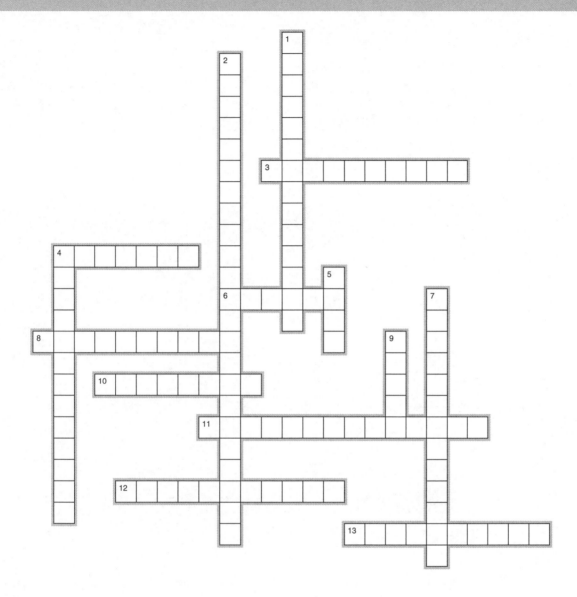

Across

3. Special imaging technique that blurs out anatomy outside the plane of interest using tube motion
4. Determines the level of the object plane in linear tomography
6. Measured using lp/mm
8. Type of distortion that makes an image appear longer than the actual object
10. Direction of tube angulation toward the head
11. Type of distortion that makes an image appear shorter than the actual object
12. An example of involuntary motion
13. Change in image size or shape

Down

1. States that any combination of mA and time with the same mAs will produce the same density or exposure
2. Exam that uses a pencil beam of x-rays to check the bony trabeculae for signs of osteoporosis
4. The primary controlling factor of detail
5. Patient motion may cause this; opposite of detail
7. Change in image size
9. Snowy appearance of an image if there is an inadequate number of photons covering the image receptor

12

Grids and Scatter Reduction

1. Increasing the field size will _____ the amount of scatter.

   a. increase
   b. decrease
   c. not change

2. Increasing the x-ray beam energy will _____ the amount of scatter.

   a. increase
   b. decrease
   c. not change

3. A decrease in patient thickness will _____ the amount of scatter.

   a. increase
   b. decrease
   c. not change

4. Most of the scattered radiation reaching the film during an x-ray exposure has an energy

   a. greater than the primary beam
   b. equal to that of the primary beam
   c. less than that of the primary beam
   d. equal to 1.02 MeV or above

5. The grid ratio is the ratio of the

   a. height of the lead strips to the distance between the lead strips
   b. height of the lead strips to the width of the lead strips
   c. height of the plastic strips to the width of the plastic strips
   d. thickness of the grid to the width of the cassette

6. A grid should usually be employed in which of the following circumstances?

   1. When radiographing a large or dense body part
   2. When using high kVp
   3. When less patient dose is required

   a. 1 and 2 only
   b. 2 and 3 only
   c. 3 only
   d. 1, 2, and 3

7. The undesirable reduction of density on one or both sides of a radiograph due to misalignment of the x-ray beam to a grid is called

   a. primary beam scatter
   b. grid cutoff
   c. grid frequency
   d. grid fog

8. Grid cutoff can result from

   a. a focused grid used at the wrong SID
   b. using small SIDs with a parallel grid
   c. an upside-down focused grid
   d. all of the above

9. A grid is designed with lead strips 0.5 mm apart. The height of the lead strips is 8 mm. What is the grid ratio?

   a. 16:1
   b. 8:1
   c. 12:1
   d. 10:1

10. When a grid with a higher grid ratio is used, the radiation dose to the patient will _____ and the radiographic contrast will _____.

    a. increase; decrease
    b. increase; increase
    c. decrease; increase
    d. decrease; decrease

11. When an 8:1 grid ratio is replaced with a 16:1 grid,

    a. the mAs must be increased
    b. the mAs must be decreased
    c. the radiographic contrast is unchanged
    d. none of the above

12. The use of grids has no effect on

    a. image contrast
    b. scatter radiation cleanup
    c. x-ray beam energy
    d. image gray scale

A radiographic examination using a focused grid produces images with densities that are lighter toward the edges. Questions 13 through 17 list various factors as possible causes. Answer a for true if the factor causes this appearance and b for false if it does not.

13. _____ Patient motion

14. _____ Incorrect SID

15. _____ Poor film/screen contact

16. _____ SID in focusing range

17. _____ Grid placed upside down

18. Which of the following are used to improve contrast and reduce scatter?

    a. collimation and filtration
    b. grids and collimation
    c. filtration and grids
    d. high kVp and long SID

19. A grid that is constructed so that all of the grid strips match the divergence of the x-ray beam would be a(n)

    a. focused grid
    b. linear grid
    c. oscillating grid
    d. crossed grid

20. Which of the following will cause an increase in film contrast?

    a. increased scatter
    b. smaller grid ratios
    c. increased grid cutoff
    d. smaller field sizes

21. An exposure made at 70 kVp and 10 mAs without a grid produces an acceptable density, but with too much scatter. A second exposure using a 12:1 grid is used. What should the new mAs be to maintain density?

    a. 2 mAs
    b. 25 mAs
    c. 50 mAs
    d. 100 mAs

22. A technique of 400 mA and 100 ms is used with a 16:1 grid. If an exam is done using a 6:1 grid, what new mAs is needed to maintain density?

    a. 2 mAs
    b. 20 mAs
    c. 0.2 mAs
    d. 200 mAs

23. The number of grid strips or grid lines per inch or centimeter is called

    a. grid ratio
    b. grid frequency
    c. line pair
    d. line focus principle

24. **A focused grid**

    a. is always used with thin body parts
    b. must be used with the correct SID
    c. requires a decrease in mAs compared to the nongrid mAs
    d. has a Bucky factor of zero

25. **The Bucky factor**

    a. indicates how much contrast will increase when comparing non-grid and grid exposures
    b. indicates how fast the grid is moving
    c. indicates how much mAs must be increased compared to non-grid techniques
    d. indicates how much scatter radiation is present

26. **A 12:1 ratio grid is substituted for an 8:1 grid. If identical technical factors are used, the new film will possess a higher**

    a. radiographic contrast
    b. radiographic density
    c. percentage of scatter
    d. all of the above

27. **Which of the following is a disadvantage of using a moving grid?**

    a. increased detail
    b. decreased SID
    c. increased OID
    d. increased grid cutoff

28. **The wall Bucky in your department is supplied with a 12:1 grid with a specified focal range of 65 to 80 in. You perform an emergency upright shoulder examination at an appropriate technique. Which of the following statements would correctly describe the appearance of the finished radiograph?**

    a. grid cutoff on one side of the image
    b. grid cutoff on all four sides of the image
    c. grid cutoff along both edges of the film
    d. density will be maintained throughout the image (i.e., no change)

29. **Which of the following interspace materials would produce a more durable grid?**

    a. lead
    b. paper
    c. wood
    d. aluminium

30. **The air gap technique is utilized to reduce scatter**

    a. with the use of a grid
    b. without the use of a grid
    c. with a short SID
    d. with air filtering out the scatter

Image Labeling

1. Label the lettered components of the diagram by illustrating the relationship of the patient, the film, and grid materials.

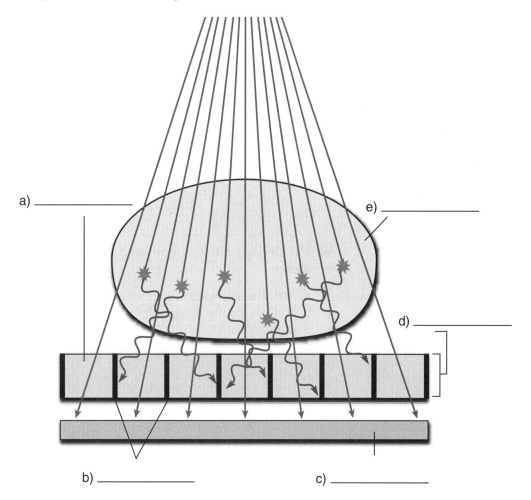

2. Label letters a through d, indicating whether the dimension shown is "height" or "distance."

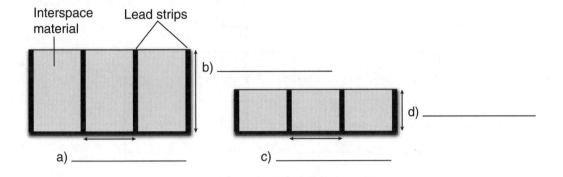

Interspace material   Lead strips

b) _____

d) _____

a) _____   c) _____

3. Complete the table by listing the appropriate Bucky factor (grid conversion factor) by each grid shown.

Grid Ratios and Associated Bucky Factors or Grid Conversion Factor

Grid Ratio	Bucky Factor or GCF
None	
5:1	
6:1	
8:1	
12:1	
16:1	

4. Describe the radiographic density that would be observed if the grid error causes listed in the second column occurred during a radiographic examination.

Grid Artifact Appearances and Their Possible Changes

Optical Density	Possible Causes
	Parallel grid at too short SID
	Upside-down focused grid
	Focused grid outside focal distance range
	Grid center not aligned with central axis
	Grid not perpendicular to central axis

Crossword Puzzle

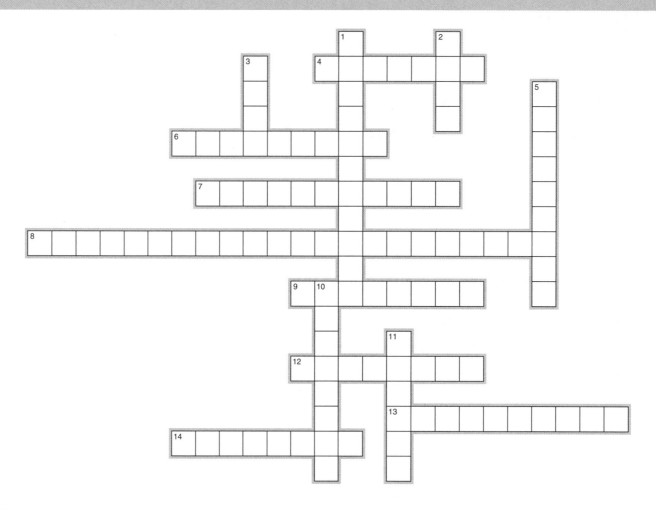

Across

4. Type of grid that must be used at a specific SID
6. Calculated using the formula: h/D
7. Circular Bucky motion
8. Device that automatically collimates to the size of the image receptor placed in the Bucky grid
9. Image quality that is the most improved when a grid is used
12. Interspace material commonly used in grid construction
13. General term for a grid error that causes a loss of density on one or both sides of an image
14. Type of grid where the lead strips are laid down in a line

Down

1. Defines the size and shape of the primary beam; used to limit field size
2. Radiopaque material used to construct a grid
3. Device made of lead strips to absorb scatter radiation
5. Number of lead strips per cm
10. Type of grid error that occurs when the grid is not perpendicular to the central ray
11. A scatter reduction technique that utilizes a large OID

PART IV

Special Imaging Techniques

Fluoroscopy, Conventional and Digital

13

1. The input phosphor of an image intensifier is coated with _____ and the output phosphor is made of _____.

   a. zinc cadmium sulfide (ZnCdS); cesium iodide (CsI)
   b. calcium tungstate (CaWO$_4$); zinc cadmium sulfide (ZnCdS)
   c. cesium iodide (CsI); zinc cadmium sulfide (ZnCdS)
   d. cesium iodide (CsI); calcium tungstate (CaWO$_4$)

2. The output phosphor of an image intensifier converts

   a. electron energy into light photons
   b. light photons into electrons
   c. light photons into x-rays
   d. electrons into x-rays

3. The electrostatic lenses of an image intensifier

   a. convert electron energy into light photons
   b. convert x-ray energy into light photons
   c. convert light photons into electrons
   d. focus electrons to converge on the output phosphor

4. The primary disadvantage of using the magnification mode rather than the standard image mode on an image intensifier is that it

   a. increases image magnification
   b. increases the patient dose
   c. produces a higher resolution image
   d. produces a brighter image

5. In an image intensifier tube, the _____ gain occurs because the input diameter is larger than the output diameter.

   a. minification
   b. confiscation
   c. flux
   d. radiation

6. _____ gain is due to the acceleration of the photoelectrons.

   a. Magnification
   b. Confiscation
   c. Flux
   d. Radiation

7. Flux gain and minification gain can be multiplied together to determine

   a. image magnification
   b. total image resolution
   c. total brightness gain
   d. automatic brightness control

8. The ABC detector automatically adjusts the

   a. attenuation of the patient
   b. input brightness of the image intensifier tube
   c. output brightness of the image intensifier tube
   d. brightness of the ambient light available

9. The ABC circuit adjusts _____ to maintain _____.

   a. constant brightness; constant mA
   b. mA; constant brightness
   c. mA; constant patient thickness
   d. patient thickness; constant brightness

10. The area of the eye where cones are concentrated is known as the

    a. lens
    b. cornea
    c. retina
    d. iris

11. The _____ in the eye are used for viewing in dim light.

    a. rods
    b. cones
    c. optic discs
    d. olfactory bulbs

12. One of the advantages of image intensification is that it

    a. increases patient dose
    b. allows cone vision to be used
    c. increases the likelihood of quantum mottle
    d. allows vignetting to occur

13. Fluoroscopic mA currents are in the range from

    a. 0.5 to 5 mA
    b. 50 to 100 mA
    c. 100 to 200 mA
    d. 300 to 400 mA

14. The minimum distance between the source and the patient's skin surface for a fixed fluoroscopic unit is ____ cm.

    a. 15
    b. 30
    c. 38
    d. 42

15. The fluoroscopic timer must have an audible signal that is heard when _____ minutes of fluoroscopy time has elapsed.

    a. 2
    b. 5
    c. 10
    d. 15

16. Fluoroscopy is utilized to observe moving structures in the body. This is termed

    a. static imaging
    b. dynamic imaging
    c. magnification imaging
    d. spot film imaging

17. Image intensification is consistently used as an accessory device for fluoroscopy. Its primary purpose is to

    a. allow more than one person to view the image at one time
    b. increase the brightness levels of the original image
    c. reduce patient skin dose
    d. shorten overall exam time

18. When the output image is digitized and continuously displayed on the TV monitor, this is known as

    a. last image hold
    b. magnification
    c. automatic brightness control
    d. brightness gain

19. Which of the following devices is responsible for converting the light image from the output phosphor into an electric signal?

    a. beam-splitting mirror
    b. input phosphor
    c. cathode ray tube (CRT)
    d. TV camera

20. An intensifier has a flux gain of 45 and a minification gain of 230. Determine the total brightness gain for this unit.

    a. 26
    b. 275
    c. 2,025
    d. 10,350

21. An image intensifier has the following dimensions: input phosphor = 12 cm and output phosphor = 3.5 cm. Compute and select the minifaction gain below.

    a. 15.5
    b. 11.8
    c. 8.5
    d. 3.4

22. A particular image intensifier tube has a flux gain of 75. The diameter of the input phosphor is 15 cm and the diameter of the output phosphor is 3 cm. The total gain for this image intensifier tube is about

    a. 375
    b. 1,125
    c. 1,875
    d. 18,750

23. What is the device that directs the light emitted from the image intensifier to various viewing and imaging apparatus?

    a. spot film changer
    b. output phosphor
    c. beam splitter
    d. automatic brightness control

24. The input phosphor of an image intensifier is responsible for converting

    a. x-rays to light
    b. x-rays to electrons
    c. light to electrons
    d. electrons to light

25. Which of the following factors would affect quantum mottle the most?

    a. OID
    b. focal point position
    c. minification geometry
    d. tube mA

26. Federal requirements limit total fluoroscopy tube output to

    a. 5,000 mrem/y
    b. 10 R/min
    c. 100 mR/h
    d. 1 R/day at 1 m

27. Which of the following devices contain an electron gun?

    1. Vidicon camera tube
    2. CRT
    3. Image intensifier tube

    a. 1 and 2
    b. 1 and 3
    c. 2 and 3
    d. 1, 2, and 3

28. Reduced image brightness on the periphery of a fluoroscopy image due to the concave shape of the input phosphor is called

    a. vignetting
    b. flicker
    c. distortion
    d. mottling

29. The _____ pattern used by the video camera tube or CCD creates the lines of one TV frame.

    a. photopic
    b. photoelectron
    c. raster
    d. cathode ray

30. In order to eliminate flicker,

    a. the CCD is connected to the output phosphor using fiber optics
    b. the target is coated with cesium antimony
    c. the video signal is doubled when ABC is activated
    d. the electron beam scans only ½ the frame at a time, and more frames per second are projected

Image Labeling

1. Identify the lettered components of the image intensifier tube.

a) _____
b) _____
c) _____
d) _____
   _____
   _____
e) _____
f) _____

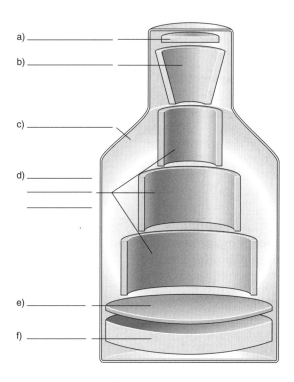

2. Trace the energy conversions that occur when an image intensifier tube is operated (letters a through d). For letters e through g, indicate the electrostatic charge that is present in that portion of the image intensifier tube.

Conversions   **Parts (Charge)**

d) _____

Focal point _____

c) _____
   _____

b) _____

a) _____

Output phosphor
Anode g) _____
Glass envelope
f) _____
e) _____
Input phosphor

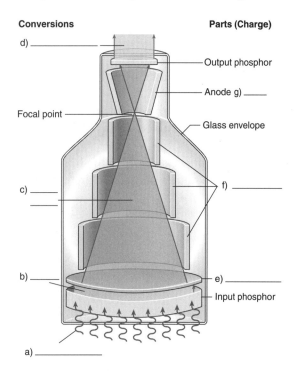

3. Label components a to j for the video camera tube shown.

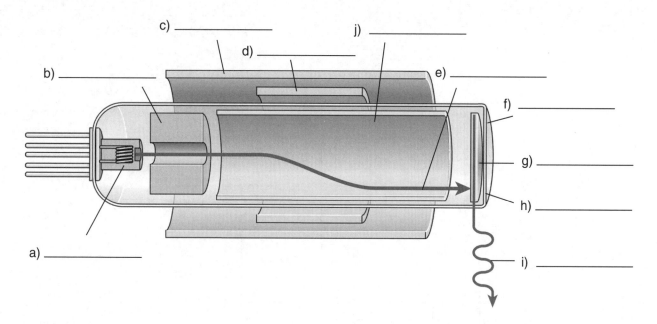

c) _____   j) _____

d) _____

b) _____   e) _____

f) _____

g) _____

h) _____

a) _____

i) _____

4. Identify the lettered components a to k of the CRT.

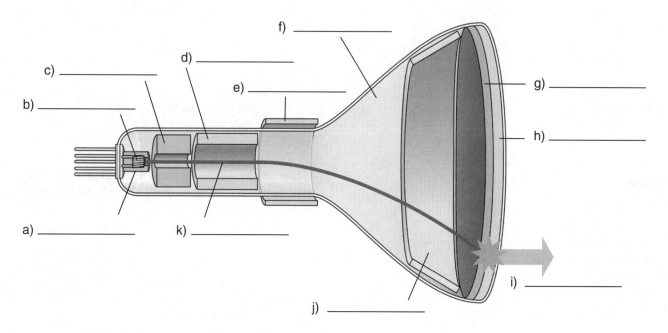

f) _____

d) _____

c) _____   e) _____

b) _____   g) _____

h) _____

a) _____   k) _____

i) _____

j) _____

Crossword Puzzle

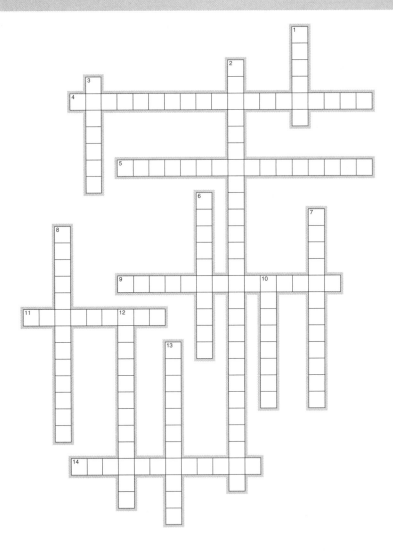

Across

4. Function to accelerate and focus the photoelectrons toward the output phosphor
5. Component of a fluoroscopic unit responsible for brightening the image
9. Composed of zinc cadmium sulfide; component of image intensifier that converts electrons to light
11. The type of video camera tube with the fastest response time
14. Type of brightness gain that results due to difference in size between the input and output phosphors

Down

1. The type of pattern created in the video camera tube by the electron beam's back and forth scanning path

2. Maintains image density and contrast at a constant level by changing tube output when patient thickness changes
3. Seen on the TV screen if the image frame rate is too slow
6. Loss of brightness at the periphery of the image due to the concave surface of the input phosphor
7. Component of an image intensifier, which converts light photons to electrons
8. Grainy appearance of an image due to an insufficient number of photons
10. Type of vision used in dim light due to the activation of the rods in the eye
12. Phosphor in the image intensifier, which receives x-ray photons and converts them to light photons
13. Dynamic imaging modality used to observe moving structures in the body

Digital Imaging

14

1. A digital image is made up of

   a. a pixel of matrices
   b. a matrix of pixels
   c. a vortex of pixels
   d. a matrix of vortices

2. Which matrix size has the smallest pixels?

   a. 128 × 128
   b. 256 × 256
   c. 512 × 512
   d. 1,024 × 1,024

3. What is the pixel size in millimeters of a 256 matrix with a 25-cm field of view (FOV)?

   a. 0.1
   b. 1.0
   c. 10
   d. 100

4. What is the pixel size in millimeters of a 512 matrix with a 30-cm FOV?

   a. 0.06
   b. 0.6
   c. 6.0
   d. 60

5. What is the pixel size in millimeters of a 256 matrix with a 15-cm FOV?

   a. 0.06
   b. 0.6
   c. 6.0
   d. 60

6. The FOV best describes

   a. the number of pixels in a matrix
   b. the imaging plane that is best demonstrated
   c. how much of the patient is imaged in a matrix
   d. the use of multiformat cameras to display multiple images

7. If the FOV remains unchanged and the matrix size increases, the spatial resolution will be

   a. improved
   b. degraded

8. Which of the following will allow more line pairs per millimeter to be imaged?

   a. using a smaller matrix
   b. increasing the number of pixels
   c. increasing the bit depth
   d. using a higher frequency signal

9. **The number of shades of gray that can be demonstrated in a digital image is affected by**

   a. matrix size
   b. bit depth
   c. FOV
   d. data compression

10. **Contrast resolution describes**

    a. the maximum separation of two objects that can be distinguished as separate objects on the image
    b. the minimum density difference between two tissues that can distinguish separate tissues
    c. the maximum density difference between two tissues that can be distinguished as separate tissues
    d. the minimum separation of two objects that can be distinguished as separate objects on the image

11. **The window width control is used to alter image**

    a. contrast
    b. density (brightness)
    c. signal-to-noise ratio
    d. resolution

12. **The window level control is used to alter image**

    a. contrast
    b. density (brightness)
    c. resolution
    d. signal-to-noise ratio

13. **An advantage of PACS is that it allows images to be**

    a. stored in hard copy format
    b. saved to prevent image manipulation after exposure
    c. sent to several workstations and monitors simultaneously
    d. created using film and automatic processing

14. **Dry film processors**

    a. use dry chemicals to produce the image
    b. use holding magazines that must be loaded in a darkroom
    c. use heat to produce the image
    d. use fragile detector plates

15. **Which of the following layers in a computed radiography cassette serves to ground the plate and reduce static electricity?**

    a. conductive layer
    b. phosphor layer
    c. protective layer
    d. light shield layer

16. **Data compression**

    a. results in faster processing
    b. produces faster transmission times
    c. requires less storage space
    d. does all of the above

17. **Direct radiography eliminates the need for the _____ because the image is captured by multiple sensors that create an image signal immediately.**

    a. image receptor cassette
    b. monitor
    c. automatic brightness control
    d. photomultiplier tube

18. **In order to view a digital image that has been exposed on a phosphor plate cassette, what "processing" equipment is needed?**

    a. a conventional daylight processor
    b. a barcode-enabled RIS
    c. a radiographic film scanner
    d. a laser reader

19. **Spatial detail in a digital imaging system would be improved the MOST by**

    a. increasing the window width
    b. decreasing the window level
    c. increasing the number of pixels
    d. decreasing the flux gain of the photomultiplier tube

20. **The "latent image" in a CR imaging plate is stored by the**

    a. photomultiplier tube
    b. analog-to-digital converter
    c. sensitivity speck
    d. trapped electrons in the phosphor center

21. In direct radiology, remnant radiation is converted into an electric signal by

    a. barium fluorohalide crystals
    b. an electron gun
    c. magnesium oxide
    d. amorphous selenium

22. The set of computer standards used to permit a wide range of digital imaging systems to ensure that images taken at one facility are able to be viewed correctly at another facility is termed

    a. DICOM
    b. PACS
    c. PSP
    d. TFT

23. If a pixel has a bit depth of 8, this means that the pixel

    a. is able to resolve 8 lp/mm
    b. can produce 2^8 shades of gray
    c. size is 0.8 mm
    d. contains 8 bytes of information

24. The algorithmic formula used to process a digital image's raw data is selected by the technologist when she/he

    a. selects the appropriate technique (mAs and kVp) on the control panel
    b. changes the FOV on the monitor
    c. alters the window level control on the monitor
    d. selects the anatomy and projection at a laser reader/workstation

25. If the signal-to-noise ratio is too low,

    a. spatial resolution is decreased
    b. the image will not be able to be compressed
    c. image contrast will be degraded
    d. the ability to use the window level and width controls is severely limited

26. The active layer in the photostimulable phosphor of a CR imaging plate is typically made of

    a. calcium tungstate
    b. rare earth materials
    c. amorphous selenium
    d. barium fluorohalide

27. The component of a direct flat panel detector that is responsible for absorbing electrons and generating the subsequent electrical charges to the image processor is the

    a. photostimulable phosphor
    b. thin-film transistor
    c. light shield layer
    d. conductive layer

28. Which device is required in order to convert a conventional radiographic film to a digital image?

    a. laser reader
    b. thermal printer head
    c. film digitizer
    d. multiformat camera

29. The device that converts the light emitted by an exposed PSP in a processing reader to an electric signal is the

    a. photomultiplier tube
    b. scanning laser
    c. thin-film transistor
    d. digital-to-analog converter

30. Before a computed radiography imaging plate can be reused, it must be

    a. stored in a darkened room for 24 hours
    b. erased with high-intensity light
    c. scanned with an electron gun
    d. recharged

Image Labeling

1. Complete the table by describing the relationships among FOV, matrix size, pixel size, and spatial resolution.

FOV	Matrix Size	Pixel Size	Spatial Resolution
Increases			
Decreases			
Remains constant			
Remains constant			

2. Label each component in the digital imaging chain.

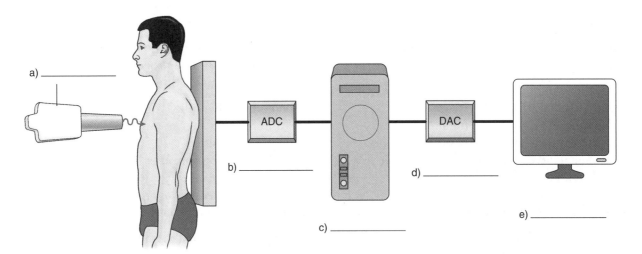

3. Identify the layers of the photostimulable phosphor.

a) _____

_____

b) _____

c) _____

d) _____

e) _____

f) _____

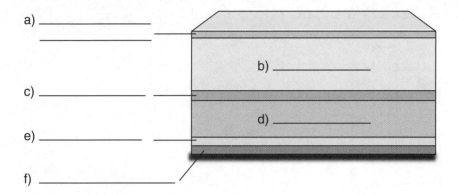

4. Identify each layer of the flat panel detector.

a) _____

b) _____

_____

c) _____

d) _____

_____

e) _____

_____

f) _____

_____

g) _____

Signal out

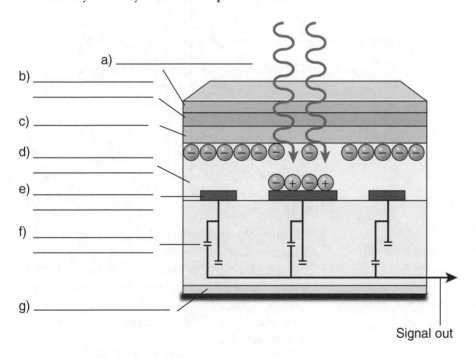

Crossword Puzzle

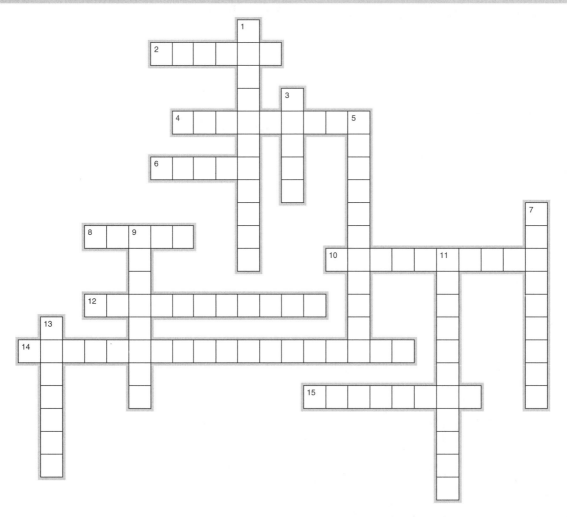

Across

2. 1,024 × 1,024 is a measure of this

4. A mathematical formula assigned to each anatomical part to create a digital image using the raw pixel data

6. Each cell in a matrix; derived from the two words, picture element

8. The type of light beam used in a CR processing reader

10. The layer in a computed radiography cassette that grounds the plate

12. Describes how much of the patient is imaged in a digital image matrix

14. A photosensitive array in a DR detector that stores electrons (charge); usually comprised of silicon

15. Digital image quality controlled by window width

Down

1. Adjusting this up or down changes the density (brightness) of a digital image

3. Acronym for the computer software standards that permit digital imaging programs to communicate with each other

5. Type of camera used to produce multiple images on a single hard copy

7. The _____ data are the raw data to which the algorithmic formula is applied to create a digital image

9. Type of semiconducting material used as a radiation conversion material in a DR flat panel detector

11. Process used to reduce the size of the data in a digital image to speed transmission times and decrease image storage space

13. Type of film used in a dry film processor

Quality Control

15

1. The sum of the difference between the light and the x-ray field edges must be within _____ of the SID.

   a. 1%
   b. 2%
   c. 5%
   d. 10%

2. The _____ can be used to measure CT spatial resolution.

   a. pinhole camera
   b. optical densitometer
   c. spinning top
   d. line pair test pattern

3. The _____ measures the size of the focal spot.

   a. pinhole camera
   b. optical densitometer
   c. spinning top
   d. bar phantom

4. The kVp of the beam should be within (±) _____ kVp of the kVp setting.

   a. 2
   b. 4
   c. 5
   d. 10

5. The penetrability or filtration of an x-ray beam is reported in terms of its

   a. EMG
   b. RTV
   c. HVL
   d. MAQ

6. The same mAs values achieved with several different mA and time settings must produce the same radiation output within _____ percent of the average.

   a. ±2
   b. ±5
   c. ±10
   d. ±20

7. A quality control program includes

   1. Periodic testing of equipment
   2. Acceptance testing
   3. Correcting deviations from expected equipment performance

   a. 1 and 2
   b. 1 and 3
   c. 2 and 3
   d. 1, 2, and 3

8. During the exposure linearity test, the mR/mAs should vary by no more than ± _____ percent from the average.

   a. 2
   b. 5
   c. 7
   d. 10

9. Mammography quality control requirements are specified in the

   a. RSNA
   b. LSMFT
   c. DDT
   d. MQSA

10. During the daily CT quality control procedure, the CT number of water is set to

    a. −1,000
    b. 0
    c. +500
    d. +1,000

11. In this series of four different exposures, which mA station does not meet the exposure linearity criteria?

    a. 50 mA, 3.2mR/mAs
    b. 100 mAs, 5.8 mR/mAs
    c. 200 mAs, 6.0 mR/mAs
    d. 400 mAs, 6.2 mR/mAs

12. The base fog density should not vary more than _____ OD from day to day.

    a. 0.01
    b. 0.05
    c. 0.1
    d. 0.2

13. According to the data below, would the radiographic unit being tested meet the federal guidelines for reproducibility? Exposure no. 1 has a machine output (mR) of 246, no. 2 – 210, no. 3 – 239, no. 4 – 259, and no. 5 – 250.

    a. yes, it is within the accuracy guidelines
    b. no, it is outside the accuracy guidelines
    c. not enough information to tell the accuracy guidelines
    d. reproducibility is not a standard QC test for mA stations

14. For optimum radiation protection, lead aprons and thyroid shields should be checked

    a. semiannually, using a resolution test tool
    b. annually, under fluoro, or exposing on a 14 × 17 cassette
    c. annually, using a water phantom
    d. semiannually, placing the apron over an R-meter

15. Processor daily sensitometric readings are limited to which of the following image function measurements?

    a. base + fog, speed, and contrast
    b. contrast, resolution, and density
    c. density, distortion, and fog
    d. magnification, temperature, and base + fog

16. A radiograph comes out of the processor with numerous dark, tree-like markings. These most likely are caused by

    a. acute bending of the film
    b. static electricity
    c. the safelight
    d. water on the loading bench

17. Any unwanted component of a radiographic image is called a(n)

    a. artifact
    b. fog
    c. plus (+) density
    d. minus (−) density

18. If dust particles or hair became trapped inside an imaging plate, the resulting artifact would be classified as which of the following?

    a. plus (+)
    b. minus (−)
    c. processor
    d. nonstochastic

19. An AP abdomen film taken on a 14 × 17 film has lines running lengthwise along it (perpendicular to the direction of film travel in the processor) at even intervals. Which of the causes below BEST explains this artifact?

    a. grid lines
    b. misaligned guide shoes
    c. pi marks
    d. backboard

20. Which of the following processor maintenance activities should be performed daily?

    a. drain and clean the deep racks
    b. clean the crossover racks
    c. fixer retention
    d. darkroom/safelight fog test

21. Which of the following would be classified as an exposure artifact?

    a. guide-shoe marks
    b. static
    c. light spots
    d. patient jewelry

22. Which of the following artifacts is most likely to result if a computed radiography imaging plate was incompletely erased?

    a. phantom images
    b. negative densities
    c. dichroic staining
    d. light spots

23. The maximum exposure rate for a fluoroscopic unit is

    a. ±5% of the first day tested
    b. 10 R/min
    c. 5 R/y
    d. ±10% of the highest mA setting

24. To ensure that the fulcrum level is accurate on a tomographic unit, a(n) _____ test should be performed.

    a. lead mask and pinhole
    b. resolution test pattern
    c. section depth indicator
    d. exposure reproducibility

25. Which of the following tests would not be appropriate to check an automatic exposure control (AEC) system?

    a. ion chamber sensitivity
    b. reproducibility
    c. backup timer verification
    d. laser localizer

26. If a viewbox in a department fails the ±10% light intensity test, what solution should be implemented?

    a. adjust the ABC density control accordingly
    b. replace the lightbulb so that the brightness is increased
    c. reduce the ambient light level so that less light interference occurs
    d. replace all of the bulbs in the viewbox bank with the same lot number

27. If the x-ray field is smaller than that indicated by the indicator knob on the collimator, a technologist risks

    a. excessive patient exposure
    b. excessive density on the radiograph
    c. cutting off anatomy of interest
    d. a nonexposed (or blank) film

28. Quality control standards require that the exposure time must be _____ from what is set.

    a. ±5%
    b. ±10%
    c. ±2%
    d. ±10 ms

29. Which of the following tools would be appropriate to conduct a filtration or HVL QC test?

    a. pinhole camera
    b. spinning top
    c. aluminum sheets
    d. metallic markers

30. If a computed radiography imaging phosphor becomes cracked or scratched, leaving minus density artifacts on the radiograph, which of the following actions should be taken to solve this problem?

    a. use the window and level functions to correct the minus densities
    b. clean the phosphor using only the appropriate solution
    c. re-erase the plate in the laser reader
    d. replace the entire phosphor in the imaging plate

Image Labeling

1. Complete the table by identifying the frequency, acceptance limits, and the test tool required for each equipment quality control test.

Factor	Monitoring Frequency	Limits	Test Tool
1. Focal spot size			
2. Spatial resolution			
3. Collimation			
4. kVp			
5. Filtration			
6. Exposure time			
7. Exposure reproducibility			
8. Exposure linearity			
9. AEC			

2. Evaluate the radiographs and identify the type of artifact density illustrated (plus or minus). For each radiograph, also determine the category(ies) of each artifact based on its cause. NOTE: Some figures may have more than one type of artifact.

a) Type of artifact density: _____

b) Artifact category(ies): _____

a) Type of artifact density: _____

b) Artifact category(ies): _____

a) Type of artifact density: _____

b) Artifact category(ies): _____

a) Type of artifact density: _____

b) Artifact category(ies): _____

Crossword Puzzle

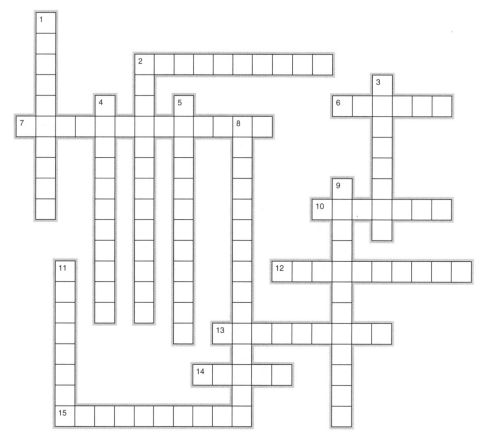

Across

2. QC test tool used to check viewbox illumination
6. This type of artifact results due to inadequate levels of humidity in the darkroom
7. This artifact appears as long lines of negative densities and is often a result of a poorly seated crossover rack
10. Noise and uniformity testing in CT rely on the use of a water _____
12. This is measured in millimeters aluminum and is derived by determining an x-ray beam's HVL
13. This measure is used to show that the radiation output of a machine is proportional to any increase or decrease in mAs
14. How frequently the temperature of the developer in the processor should be checked?
15. One of the QC tests used to check the operation of this type of unit is the section depth indicator test

Down

1. This term describes the proper alignment of the light field and the x-ray field
2. This QC test tool is used to check for the accuracy of the focal spot size
3. Examples of this class of artifacts include crease marks, static, and light leaks
4. This test determines the response of each ion chamber in an AEC device; each chamber must respond within ±10% of each other
5. This QC test tool creates a step wedge exposure on a film for processor monitoring
8. This satisfaction of this QC test demonstrates that the x-ray unit is able to produce the same radiation output (in mR) within a ±5% range when using the same technical factors
9. An artifact unique to computed radiography; caused by incomplete erasure
11. Any unwanted density or information on a radiograph

Mammography

16

1. Mammography units must have a half value layer greater than

   a. 2.50 mm molybdenum
   b. 2.50 mm aluminum
   c. 0.03 mm molybdenum
   d. 0.3 mm aluminum

2. The _____ of a mammographic x-ray tube is placed toward the chest wall to take advantage of the heel effect.

   a. cathode
   b. anode

3. Typical focal spot sizes for mammography tubes are

   a. 0.01 and 0.03 mm
   b. 0.1 and 0.3 mm
   c. 1 and 3 mm
   d. 10 and 20 mm

4. The K characteristic x-rays from a molybdenum anode tube have energies of _____ and _____ keV.

   a. 15.4; 17.9
   b. 17.4; 19.9
   c. 19.4; 21.9
   d. none of the above

5. The kVp range used for mammography is

   a. 20 to 25 kVp
   b. 20 to 40 kVp
   c. 40 to 50 kVp
   d. 60 to 90 kVp

6. Changing the kVp in a mammographic unit will _____ the energy of the K characteristic x-rays.

   a. decrease
   b. increase
   c. cause no change in

7. Extended processing of mammographic films

   a. decreases contrast
   b. decreases latitude
   c. increases patient dose
   d. decreases speed

8. A routine screening mammography examination includes _____ projections of the breast.

   1. Craniocaudal
   2. Mediolateral
   3. Lateral medial
   4. Anterior posterior

   a. 1 and 2
   b. 1 and 3
   c. 1 and 4
   d. 2 and 4

9. Magnification mammography

   a. uses the 0.3-mm focal spot
   b. is used during screening examinations
   c. is used to examine suspicious areas
   d. is accomplished by decreasing the OID

10. The average radiation dose to each breast from a typical screening examination in the United States is

    a. 1.4 mGy (140 mrad)
    b. 2.8 mGy (280 mrad)
    c. 4.5 mGy (450 mrad)
    d. 6.3 mGy (630 mrad)

11. The federal requirements for facilities and technologists who perform mammography are outlined by/in

    a. NCRP Report no. 116
    b. ACR Publication 1987
    c. the MQSA
    d. the FDA Health Advisory Report

12. The advantages of breast compression during mammography include

    1. The ability to use higher kVp
    2. Decreased patient dose
    3. Reduced magnification

    a. 1 and 2
    b. 1 and 3
    c. 2 and 3
    d. 1, 2, and 3

13. The best grid ratio for producing optimal mammographic images would be

    a. 4:1
    b. 8:1
    c. 12:1
    d. 16:1

14. Which of the following mammography unit components would most likely be constructed of beryllium?

    a. compression device
    b. port
    c. anode
    d. image receptor

15. When would a rhodium filter be preferable to a molybdenum filter?

    a. for patients whose breasts are extremely dense
    b. when magnification views are needed
    c. if federal HVL requirements are not met using only molybdenum
    d. for filmless mammography applications

16. The SID used for mammography is usually

    a. 12 to 20 in
    b. 24 to 30 in
    c. 36 to 40 in
    d. 60 to 72 in

17. The steeper anode angle of 22 to 24 degrees used on mammography units helps to ensure

    a. lower breast dose
    b. that the image contrast is increased
    c. that the magnification is reduced
    d. that the full image receptor size is covered

18. The advantage of using a molybdenum target rather than a tungsten target in mammography is that

    a. the energies of the photons produced are more conducive for differential absorption in the breast
    b. an increased number of photons are produced
    c. greater photon energies result in less tissue absorption and decreased patient dose
    d. smaller effective focal spot sizes can be achieved, resulting in better detail

19. During mammography, the AEC detector is placed

    a. between the port and the breast
    b. between the breast and the image receptor
    c. behind the image receptor
    d. above the compression device

20. In film-screen mammography, single emulsion film is generally used to

    a. decrease patient dose
    b. improve image detail
    c. correlate the image with a charged couple device
    d. increase light blur on the edge of structures

21. In order to meet federal requirements, mammography imaging systems must be able to achieve a minimum of _____ lp/mm.

    a. 2 to 4
    b. 8 to 9
    c. 11 to 13
    d. 16 to 18

22. Magnification views of the breast are achieved by

    a. increasing the OID
    b. decreasing the SID
    c. changing to a larger filament size
    d. using double emulsion film

23. The advantages of digital mammography over conventional film-screen mammography are

    1. The ability to immediately send images to remote sites
    2. Less storage space is needed for images
    3. Reduced breast dose

    a. 1 and 2
    b. 1 and 3
    c. 2 and 3
    d. 1, 2, and 3

24. Which type of digital imaging mammography system allows the breast to be scanned with both the detector and the x-ray beam in unison?

    a. computed radiography
    b. selenium flat panel
    c. phosphor CCD
    d. gadolinium oxysulfide

25. In a flat panel mammography system, the material that converts remnant x-ray photons into an electric charge is typically

    a. cesium iodide
    b. selenium
    c. thallium
    d. silver halide

26. One primary disadvantage of conducting magnification views of the breast is

    a. increased patient dose
    b. the need to create an increased SID
    c. that they are difficult to obtain using flat panel detectors
    d. difficulty aligning the AEC detector with the x-ray tube

27. The amount of force applied to the breast during compression is between _____ lb.

    a. 4 and 5
    b. 10 and 20
    c. 25 and 45
    d. 50 and 75

28. Microcalcifications in the breast are best evaluated using a

    a. high-contrast image
    b. low-resolution image
    c. large focal spot size
    d. double-emulsion film

29. The purpose of an AEC system in a mammography unit is to

    a. ensure proper centering and compression of the breast
    b. terminate the exposure when the proper dose to the detector is reached
    c. increase the total filtration to the required mm/Al equivalent
    d. allow fiber optics to be employed when converting to digital mammography

30. In computed radiography of the breast, the image is captured by

    a. silver halide crystals in the emulsion
    b. amorphous selenium
    c. cesium iodide phosphors
    d. energy traps in an imaging plate

Image Labeling

1. Identify the anatomy of the breast shown.

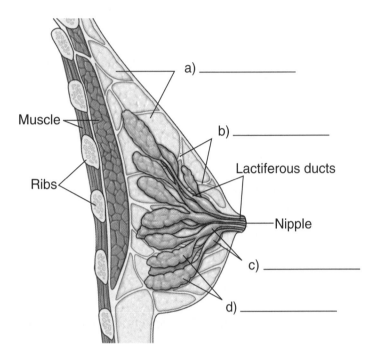

2. Label each lettered component of a dedicated mammography unit.

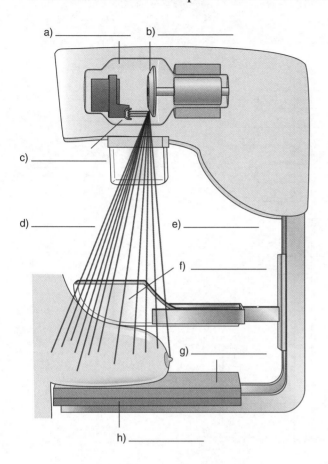

3. Label the diagram, identifying each layer of a mammography film-screen cassette.

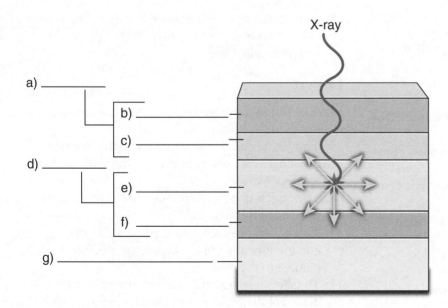

Crossword Puzzle

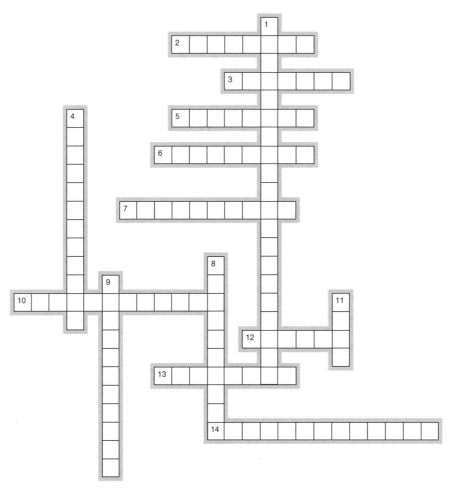

Across

2. This image quality is improved when grids are used
3. This type of filter may be used for patients with extremely dense breasts
5. Most flat panel digital detectors are constructed of this material
6. The port of the mammography tube is often constructed of this material
7. The maximum amount should not exceed 0.4 mm aluminum equivalent
10. This routine mammography projection directs the central ray inferiorly from the patient's head to the feet
12. The best image detail of the breast would be created using _____ emulsion film
13. This describes the type of processing used when film processing time is increased

14. This imaging technique is used to examine suspicious areas of the breast and is accomplished by increasing the OID

Down

1. A common rare earth screen phosphor used in mammography cassettes
4. This term is used to describe the filament when one single filament is used for both small and large focal spot sizes
8. The targets of most mammography units are constructed of this material
9. This plastic device is mounted on a mammographic unit and applies an average of 25 to 45 lb of force to the breast
11. To take advantage of this effect, the cathode is placed at the patient's chest wall and the anode is placed toward the nipple

Computed Tomography

17

1. An x-ray tube in a CT scanner has

   a. two cathodes
   b. a high heat capacity
   c. a molybdenum anode
   d. a stationary anode

2. The thickness of a CT slice is controlled by the

   a. target angle
   b. filament size
   c. patient thickness
   d. adjustable collimators

3. A voxel is

   a. a picture element
   b. a volume element
   c. a data storage element
   d. the pixels arranged in columns and rows

4. Detectors used in CT scanners are

   a. solid state
   b. gas filled
   c. scintillation
   d. all of the above

5. The crystal of choice in current CT scintillation detectors is

   a. sodium iodide
   b. xenon
   c. cadmium tungstate
   d. carbon graphite

6. The patient support table

   a. is made of low attenuation material
   b. is portable and may be used for patient transport
   c. has no relationship to the pitch
   d. contains the detector elements

7. Spatial resolution describes the _____ of two objects that can be distinguished as separate objects.

   a. Hounsfield unit
   b. minimum separation
   c. maximum size
   d. absorption differential

8. Contrast resolution describes the ability to distinguish the _____ of two objects.

   a. separation
   b. attenuation difference
   c. motion
   d. size

9. Indexing refers to the

   a. amount of table movement
   b. tube rotation speed
   c. rotations per centimeter of patient motion
   d. changes in high voltage

10. The computer programs or formulae that calculate the CT numbers are called

    a. Pym programs
    b. soft contrast diagrams
    c. Hounsfield units
    d. algorithms

11. The CT number of fat is

    a. −1,000
    b. −100
    c. 0
    d. 1,000

12. The CT number for bone is

    a. −1,000
    b. −50
    c. 0
    d. 1,000

13. Reverse display can be used to

    a. convert a hard copy image to an electronic version
    b. return all convoluted pixel values back to their original values
    c. change the blacks on an image to white and vice versa
    d. allow image construction in a previous scanning plane

14. In _____ CT scanning, the table moves continuously through the gantry.

    a. conventional
    b. spiral
    c. step and shoot
    d. first-generation

15. Fifth-generation CT scanning is dedicated to imaging (the)

    a. head
    b. abdominal structures
    c. cardiac system
    d. spine

16. One major advantage of CT scanning is its

    a. high count rate
    b. small pixel sizes
    c. table motion
    d. high contrast resolution

17. The breakthrough in sixth-generation CT technology that allows for the continuous motion of the patient through the gantry is the use of

    a. adjustable collimators
    b. convolution
    c. slip rings
    d. suppression

18. The scanogram taken during a CT procedure is used to

    a. annotate any special windowing used to obtain the images
    b. serve as a scout and reference guide to the section intervals taken
    c. ensure the patient is not wearing any metal objects or other artifact-causing materials
    d. check the linearity of the CT numbers of bone in the image to water

19. Which of the following will provide the greatest image spatial resolution?

    a. small pixels, small focal spot size, and narrow collimation
    b. large pixels, higher atomic numbers, and wide collimation
    c. small indexes, faster tube speeds, and large voxels
    d. small voxels, large fields of view, and limited deconvolution

20. To correct for the "cork-screw" image that results due to helical scanning, which of the following image processing tools is used?

    a. reformatting
    b. reverse image
    c. filtering and windowing
    d. interpolation

21. The component of a scintillation detector that is responsible for causing the amplification of the electrons prior to being processed by the computer is the

    a. photomultiplier tube
    b. dynode
    c. sodium iodide crystal
    d. tungsten plate

22. The collimator determines and/or controls which of the following in CT scanning?

    1. Slice thickness
    2. Patient dose
    3. Table index

    a. 1 and 2
    b. 1 and 3
    c. 2 and 3
    d. 1, 2, and 3

23. The CT calibration test that is conducted to ensure that water is consistently represented as zero Hounsfield units is called

    a. indexing
    b. deconvolution
    c. linearity
    d. line pair measure

24. Image reconstruction in CT scanning relies heavily on the use of which principle?

    a. Fourier transformation
    b. Hounsfield indexing
    c. voxel effect
    d. fan beam technology

25. A broad dark band is apparent on an abdominal CT image. This probably resulted due to

    a. the presence of metal objects in the scanning field
    b. patient motion
    c. increased beam attenuation through the patient
    d. a detector that has fallen out of calibration

26. Which of the following is most likely to cause a star artifact?

    a. beam hardening
    b. algorithm errors
    c. tissue averaging
    d. patient jewelry

27. The average radiation dose per slice during a CT scan is about

    a. 1 mGy
    b. 15 mGy
    c. 30 mGy
    d. 60 mGy

28. Modern CT scanners have x-ray beams that are

    a. pencil beams
    b. fan shaped
    c. divergent
    d. helical

29. Each pixel in a CT image is displayed as

    a. a distinct brightness level
    b. a relative attenuation value
    c. two line pairs
    d. a dotted line on a scanogram

30. If the table movement is equal to the section thickness, then the pitch is

    a. 100:1
    b. 10:1
    c. 2:1
    d. 1:1

Image Labeling

1. Identify the components of the CT scanner and the anatomy of the abdominal CT scan.

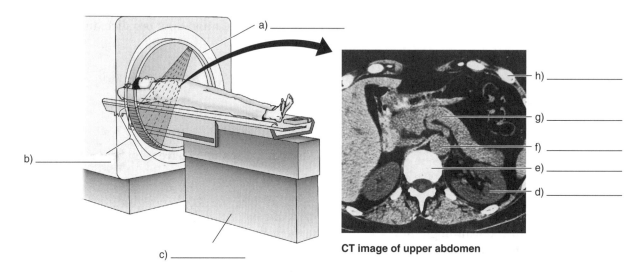

CT image of upper abdomen

2. Label the lettered components of the scintillation detector.

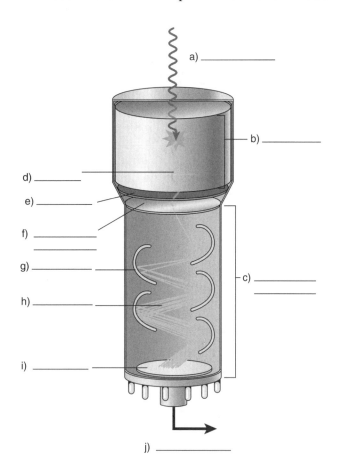

3. **Complete the table by placing the Hounsfield unit or CT number for each tissue type in the appropriate box.**

Tissue	Hounsfield Unit or CT Number
Air	
Lung	
Fat	
Water	
Tumors	
Blood	
Cerebrospinal fluid	
Gray matter	
White matter	
Muscle	
Liver	
Blood, clotted	
Dense bone	

Crossword Puzzle

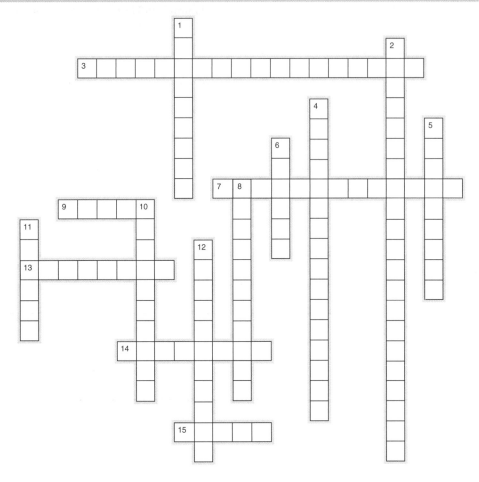

Across

3. The ability of a system to distinguish between two objects with similar attenuation values
7. This type of detector is composed of sodium iodide crystals that emit light when struck by an x-ray photon
9. The distance that the patient travels through the CT scanner; the ratio of tube movement to section thickness
13. The positioning of the table; must be reproducible within 1 mm
14. These types of objects in the body are responsible for creating star artifacts
15. The volume of each pixel element

Down

1. Term for the scout image of the area to be scanned
2. The primary mathematical method used to create the manifest image by the computer using algorithms
4. Preferred CT scintillation detector crystal due to its minimal afterglow
5. The mathematical formula/calculations performed by the computer that produces the image
6. The doughnut-shaped structure and patient aperture in a CT scanner
8. Process of modifying pixel values using mathematical formulas; applies a mask to the image
10. This unit assigns specific values to different types of tissue based on their attenuation properties
11. Sixth-generation CT scanners; allows continuous rotation of the x-ray tube and detectors around the patient
12. Term for the synchronization of the x-ray tube and detectors while scanning a patient

Magnetic Resonance Imaging

18

1. **The Larmor frequency is the resonant frequency of the**

   a. magnetic field
   b. superconducting coils
   c. protons in a magnetic field
   d. permanent magnet

2. **In MRI, resonance is the**

   a. loss of resistance of low temperatures
   b. moving of hydrogen protons in and out of alignment
   c. creation of a fringe magnetic field
   d. volume of a Dewar vessel

3. **The hydrogen protons are excited during MR imaging by**

   a. RF pulses at the Larmor resonance frequency
   b. RF pulses in the fringe field
   c. contrast material injection
   d. RF pulses outside the bore

4. **Permanent magnets**

   a. produce low fields
   b. have a wide bore
   c. require no external electrical power
   d. all of the above

5. **MR images are obtained utilizing ionizing radiation**

   a. true
   b. false

6. **Superconducting magnets**

   a. produce ionizing radiation
   b. must be maintained at very low temperatures
   c. create large amounts of electrical resistance
   d. require no special department accommodations

7. **Protons precessing back into alignment with the external magnetic field have a specific**

   a. velocity
   b. relaxation time
   c. recombination time
   d. orbital residence

8. **Hydrogen protons are useful for producing MR images because**

   a. they are the most abundant element in the body
   b. they are naturally magnetic
   c. they are not affected by a magnetic field
   d. they are electrically charged

9. **Gradient coils are used to**

   a. select the slice to be imaged
   b. produce and detect RF signals
   c. prevent excess heating during scanning
   d. improve the homogeneity of the magnetic field

10. **Liquid helium**

    a. is a superconducting liquid
    b. must be kept at temperatures above 23°C
    c. is used in permanent magnet MR units
    d. is used to cool superconducting coils

11. **A dewar is**

    a. liquid helium
    b. a vacuum container
    c. a gradient coil
    d. a superconducting coil

12. **T1 is the time associated with the**

    a. harmonic frequency bandwidth
    b. proton's loss of phase
    c. protons precessing into alignment
    d. gradient signal resonance

13. **T2 is the time**

    a. needed to turn off the magnet
    b. taken for protons to lose their phase
    c. taken for the RF signal strength to reach its peak
    d. noted for exams using contrast media

14. **The MR room is surrounded with a copper cage in order to**

    a. protect the patient from harmful electromagnetic waves
    b. generate a stronger magnetic field
    c. prevent external RF signals from entering the room
    d. shield the area outside the room from magnetic waves

15. **Surface coils are used to**

    a. select the slice to be imaged
    b. produce and detect RF signals
    c. prevent excessive heating during scanning
    d. improve the homogeneity of the magnetic field

16. **The knocking or rapping noise during MR scanning is caused by pulsing of the**

    a. magnetic coil
    b. gradient coils
    c. signal coils
    d. shim coils

17. **Precessing occurs when**

    a. the protons send out RF signals
    b. the patient is screened for metal objects prior to the MRI scan
    c. protons are brought into alignment in a magnetic field
    d. an RF excitation pulse is sent into the aligned protons

18. **What is the relationship between the magnetic field strength and Larmor frequency values?**

    a. as magnetic field strength increases, Larmor frequency increases
    b. as magnetic field strength increases, Larmor frequency decreases
    c. as magnetic field strength decreases, Larmor frequency increases
    d. no relationship exists between magnetic field strength and Larmor frequency

19. **MR images are produced from the**

    a. precessing protons while in alignment
    b. RF pulses sent by the surface coil
    c. magnetic field created by the superconducting coil
    d. RF signals exiting protons moving back into alignment

20. **The primary determining factor of MR signal strength or image brightness is**

    a. the contents of the dewar vessel
    b. proton or spin density
    c. the effectiveness of the Faraday cage
    d. proximity of the bore to the anatomy being imaged

21. **The preferred contrast material for MR imaging studies is**

    a. gadolinium DTPA
    b. liquid nitrogen
    c. barium
    d. iodinated contrast materials

22. **MR is able to produce images of all tissue types because**

    a. tissues absorb x-rays at different rates
    b. some protons are affected by magnetic fields and others are not
    c. protons in different tissues have different relaxation times
    d. RF pulses are not absorbed by the body, but simply reflected back

23. **What is the relationship between T1 and T2 relaxation times?**

    a. T1 times are always shorter than T2 times
    b. T2 times are always shorter than T1 times
    c. they are always exactly equal

24. **In order to obtain the highest image contrast, which of the following should be adjusted?**

    a. the kVp should be decreased
    b. the Faraday cage strength should be increased
    c. the part should be placed as close as possible to the magnet
    d. the RF signal strength should be set so that a large difference exists between two tissues

25. **Which of the following tissues will appear dark in a T2-weighted image?**

    a. hematoma
    b. gray matter
    c. spinal fluid
    d. epidermal

26. **Shim coils are used to**

    a. select the desired slice location and orientation
    b. enhance the uniformity of the external magnetic field
    c. send and detect RF signals
    d. protect the patient from the magnetic field

27. **If the signal to noise ratio is less than optimal, what image quality(ies) is(are) most affected?**

    a. image brightness
    b. spatial resolution
    c. motion artifacts
    d. visibility (contrast)

28. **What class of materials should never be allowed in an MR procedure room?**

    a. paramagnetic
    b. nonferromagnetic
    c. ferromagnetic
    d. insulating

29. **The inverse cube law states that magnetic field strength**

    a. is unaffected in the presence of three-dimensional objects
    b. decreases exponentially with the cube of the distance
    c. is increased exponentially with the cubic volume of the dewar
    d. falls by a factor of three for every inch of distance

30. **To prevent injuries in the MRI department, which of the following actions should be taken?**

    a. screening patients with a history of metalworking prior to all MRI scans
    b. keeping patients with pacemakers out of the area
    c. excluding patients with metal prostheses and surgical clips from MRI scanning
    d. all of the above

Image Labeling

1. Label the lettered components of the MRI unit shown.

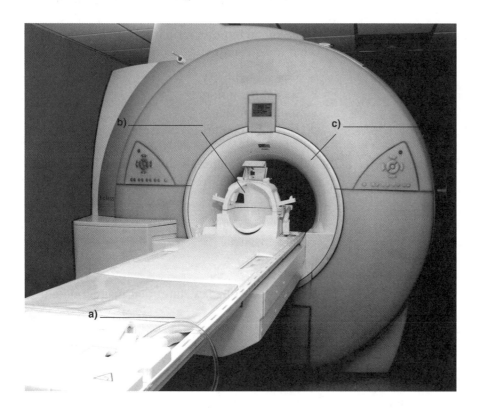

2. Identify the components of a superconducting magnet.

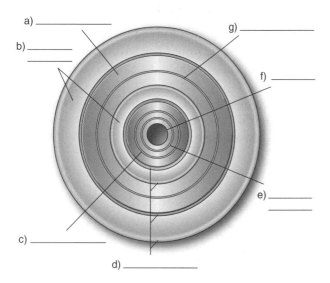

3. Identify each coil and the magnet in a typical MRI unit.

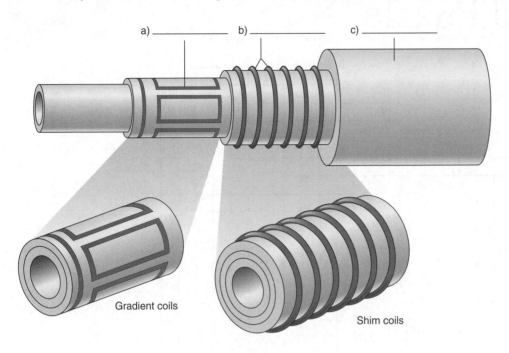

a) _____ b) _____ c) _____

Gradient coils

Shim coils

4. Complete the table, indicating whether the body tissue will appear dark or bright in a T1-weighted MR image and in a T2-weighted MR image.

The Appearance of Some Body Tissues in T1- and T2-Weighted MR Images

Body Tissue	Appearance in T1-Weighted Image	Appearance in T2-Weighted Image
White matter		
Gray matter		
Spinal fluid		
Hematoma		

Crossword Puzzle

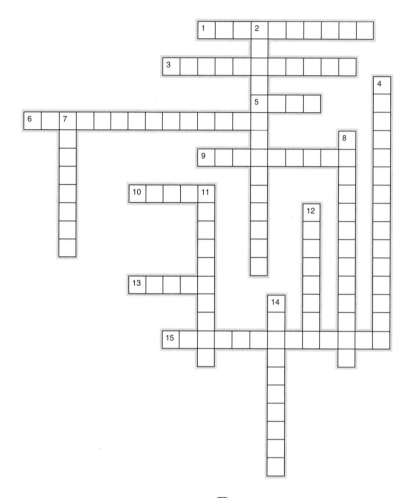

Across

1. The process that describes the alignment of spinning hydrogen atoms when in the presence of a magnetic field
3. The copper screen surrounding an MR room to block external radio frequency signals
5. The type of coil used to improve the uniformity of the magnetic field near the edges of the bore
6. Occurs when individual hydrogen nuclei spin on an axis, causing each to behave like tiny magnets
9. Moving protons in and out of alignment using magnetic fields and radio frequency pulses
10. The vacuum container that holds either liquid helium or liquid nitrogen in a superconducting MRI magnet
13. Unit used to measure magnetic strength; equal to 10,000 G
15. The quantity of hydrogen nuclei resonating in a given volume of tissue; may also be referred to as image brightness

Down

2. Fear of enclosed spaces; can be alleviated by using an open-bore MRI unit
4. The resonance value assigned to the speed of protons wobbling in a magnetic field; unique to each element in the body
7. The type of MRI coil used to select the imaging plane
8. The class of materials that are highly attracted to a magnetic field and can become projectiles in an MRI suite
11. _____ time is the time it takes for a proton to precess into alignment with a magnetic field or lose its alignment
12. The most abundant element in the human body
14. The primary component of the intravenous contrast agent preferred for MRI

PART V

Radiation Protection

19

Radiation Biology

1. The most radiosensitive part of the cell cycle is the _____ phase.

   a. S
   b. G_1
   c. M
   d. G_2

2. The least radiosensitive part of cell cycle is the _____ phase.

   a. S
   b. G_1
   c. M
   d. G_2

3. The most radioresistant tissue from the list below is

   a. lymph
   b. nerve
   c. skin
   d. thyroid

4. The Law of Bergonie and Tribondeau states that

   1. Younger cells are more radiosensitive
   2. Rapidly dividing cells are more radiosensitive
   3. Mature cells are less radiosensitive
   4. Rapidly growing cells are more radiosensitive

   a. 1 and 2
   b. 1, 2, and 4
   c. 1, 3, and 4
   d. 1, 2, 3, and 4

5. The least radioresistant cells in the human body are

   a. epithelial cells
   b. nerve cells
   c. osteocytes
   d. lymphocytes

6. The technical term for cell division of genetic cells is

   a. mitosis
   b. meiosis
   c. growth
   d. stochastic

7. The stage of high-dose radiation effects in which the individual appears to have recovered but may still exhibit symptoms at a later date is called the

   a. prodromal stage
   b. latent period
   c. acute stage
   d. recovery stage

8. The high-dose effect occurring at doses from 1 to 6 Gy (100–600 rads) is the

   a. prodromal stage
   b. hemotologic syndrome
   c. gastrointestinal syndrome
   d. central nervous syndrome

9. The high-dose effect occurring at doses from 6 to 10 Gy (300–1,000 rads) is the

   a. prodromal stage
   b. hematologic syndrome
   c. gastrointestinal syndrome
   d. central nervous syndrome

10. An indirect effect of radiation exposure to the cell involves the

   a. DNA bond
   b. cell membrane
   c. cytoplasm
   d. organelles

11. The D_Q in the cell survival curve describes the

   a. number of targets actually hit
   b. organelle damage
   c. DNA damage
   d. threshold dose of the irradiated cells

12. DNA duplication occurs during which phase of the cell cycle?

   a. prophase
   b. metaphase
   c. S phase
   d. G_1

13. It is assumed that biological effects from diagnostic radiology exposures follow the _____ dose-response model.

   a. linear threshold
   b. linear nonthreshold
   c. nonlinear threshold
   d. nonlinear nonthreshold

14. Higher doses result in _____ latent periods.

   a. shorter
   b. longer
   c. unchanged
   d. none of the above

15. Ionizing radiation is a(n)

   a. carcinogen
   b. cytoplasminogen
   c. pyrimidine
   d. organelle

16. The doubling dose for genetic effects is between _____.

   a. 0.01 and 0.1 Gy (1 and 10 rads)
   b. 0.5 and 1.0 Gy (50 and 100 rads)
   c. 2.0 and 4.0 Gy (200 and 400 rads)
   d. 5 and 10 Gy (500 and 1,000 rads)

17. Which of the following types of radiation has the highest linear energy transfer (LET)?

   a. gamma rays
   b. bremsstrahlung
   c. alpha particles
   d. x-rays

18. Immature somatic cells are called

   a. germ cells
   b. stem cells
   c. genetic cells
   d. oogonia

19. The skin erythema dose (SED 50) is approximately

   a. 50 rads (0.5 Gy)
   b. 100 rads (1 Gy)
   c. 300 rads (3 Gy)
   d. 600 rads (6 Gy)

20. The dose to produce epilation to the scalp is approximately

   a. 50 rads (0.5 Gy)
   b. 100 rads (1 Gy)
   c. 300 rads (3 Gy)
   d. 600 rads (6 Gy)

21. The $LD_{50/30}$ dose to the whole body with no medical support is approximately

   a. 50 rads (0.5 Gy)
   b. 100 rads (1 Gy)
   c. 300 rads (3 Gy)
   d. 600 rads (6 Gy)

22. The term epilation is used to refer to

   a. loss of hair
   b. lower white blood cell formation
   c. metabolism
   d. cataract formation

23. The target theory states that if ionization occurs in or near a key molecule,

    a. enzymes and proteins will be irreparably damaged
    b. restitution is still highly likely
    c. DNA may be inactivated and the cell will die
    d. two ion pairs and two free radicals are produced

24. Genetic effects of radiation are associated with

    a. RBE
    b. OER
    c. LET
    d. GSD

25. How does the LET of a radiation affect its relative biologic effectiveness (RBE)?

    a. higher LET radiations have higher RBE values
    b. higher LET radiations have lower RBE values
    c. higher LET radiations cause RBE to stabilize
    d. lower LET radiations cause RBE to stabilize

26. Cancer and genetic effects are examples of _____ effects.

    a. stochastic
    b. nonstochastic
    c. threshold
    d. acute radiation syndrome

27. Which of the following populations have experienced an excess incidence of bone cancers?

    a. uranium miners
    b. radium watch dial painters
    c. Chernobyl victims
    d. radiologic technologists

28. The stages of acute radiation syndrome in order are

    a. prodromal, latent, manifest, and recovery/death
    b. prodromal, manifest, latent, and recovery/death
    c. manifest, latent, prodromal, and recovery/death
    d. latent, manifest, prodromal, and recovery/death

29. Which of the following physiological effects are associated with and most likely to occur as a result of a patient who is a victim of the hematologic syndrome of acute radiation syndrome?

    a. decreased leukocytes and thrombocytes
    b. nausea and bloody diarrhea
    c. thrombus formation and remission
    d. headaches and coma

30. Based upon the Law of Bergonie and Tribondeau, the fetus is highly radiosensitive because of

    a. low rate of proliferation
    b. high rate of mitotic activity
    c. large numbers of mature and highly differentiated cells
    d. its environment

Image Labeling

1. Label the lettered cell components.

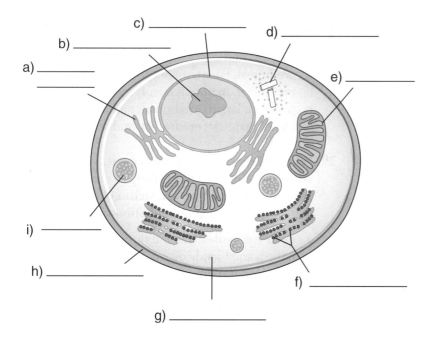

a) _____
_____

b) _____

c) _____

d) _____

e) _____

i) _____

h) _____

g) _____

f) _____

2. Complete the table by describing each step in the cell cycle.

Phase of Cell Cycle	Description
M	
G_1	
S	
G_2	

3. Identify each phase in the cell division process of mitosis.

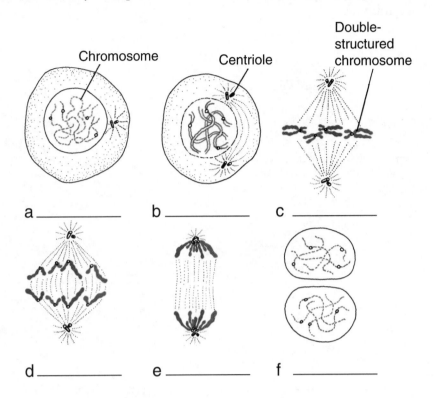

a _____   b _____   c _____

d _____   e _____   f _____

4. Label the various results due to the radiolysis of water.

H_2O

a) _____

HOH^+
HOH^-

b) _____

H^+
H^-

c) _____

OH^*
H^*

$OH^* + OH^* = H_2O_2$

d) _____

5. Complete the table by listing the cells and organs that are assigned to each category of radiosensitivity: most, intermediate, and least.

Most sensitive
_____

Intermediate
_____

Least sensitive
_____

6. **Identify the dose rate, latency period, and average time period for each syndrome associated with acute radiation syndrome.**

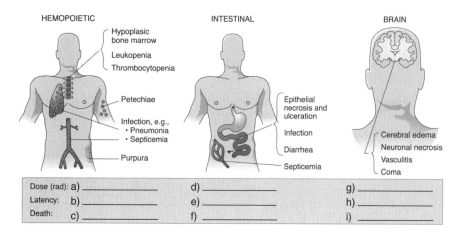

HEMOPOIETIC

- Hypoplasic bone marrow
- Leukopenia
- Thrombocytopenia
- Petechiae
- Infection, e.g.,
  - Pneumonia
  - Septicemia
- Purpura

INTESTINAL

- Epithelial necrosis and ulceration
- Infection
- Diarrhea
- Septicemia

BRAIN

- Cerebral edema
- Neuronal necrosis
- Vasculitis
- Coma

Dose (rad):	a) _____	d) _____	g) _____
Latency:	b) _____	e) _____	h) _____
Death:	c) _____	f) _____	i) _____

Crossword Puzzle

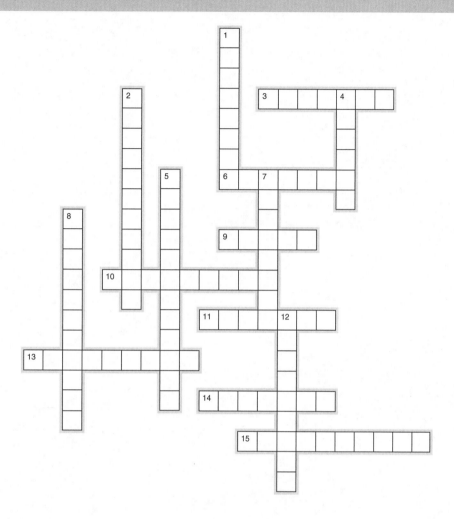

Across

3. Type of cells produced by the reproductive organs
6. The purine that pairs with thymine in a DNA molecule
9. Eighty percent of the human body is made of this substance
10. The stage of mitosis where the chromosomes are aligned across the spindle of the nucleus
11. Cataracts are an example of a late _____ effect
13. The first stage of acute radiation syndrome
14. The reduction and division process for genetic cells
15. The type of radiation effects that occur randomly; examples include cancer and genetic effects

Down

1. Cancer of the blood due to bone marrow irradiation
2. Each normal human somatic cell has 46 of these
4. This theory suggests that for a cell to die after radiation, a key molecule must be inactivated
5. Chemically reactive atoms with an unpaired electron in the outer shell that result from the radiolysis of water
7. Skin reddening due to radiation exposure
8. The ARS syndrome that occurs between 100 and 600 rads (1–6 Gy) whole body exposure; causes a decrease in leukocytes and erythrocytes
12. The minimum dose needed for a specific effect to become evident

20

Radiation Protection and Regulations

1. The primary protective barrier for fluoroscopy procedures is the

   a. lead curtain and the radiologist
   b. Bucky slot cover
   c. image intensifier
   d. patient

2. The TVL value is used to determine

   a. occupational dose
   b. adequate filtration
   c. occupancy factor
   d. primary and secondary barriers

3. By law, collimator and light field must be accurate to within

   a. ±2% of the SID
   b. ±5% of the SID
   c. ±2% of the field size
   d. ±5% of the field size

4. Which equipment performance test is used to ensure that the intensity of the output radiation remains consistent when the same exposure factors are used?

   a. exposure linearity
   b. automatic exposure
   c. filtration
   d. exposure reproducibility

5. The detector that requires heating to obtain a dose reading is the

   a. gas-filled detector
   b. scintillator
   c. TLD
   d. GM counter

6. The detector that is used to calibrate and evaluate x-ray unit performance is the

   a. gas-filled detector
   b. scintillator
   c. TLD
   d. GM counter

7. The accuracy of the source-to-image receptor distance (SID) must be

   a. ±2% of the indicated SID
   b. ±5% of the indicated SID
   c. ±10% of the indicated SID
   d. ±25% of the indicated SID

8. The type of radiation detector that gives off light when struck by radiation is a

   a. gas-filled detector
   b. GM counter
   c. scintillation detector
   d. prereading dosimeter

9. Radiation workers must wear a personnel monitor device

   1. Daily
   2. At the hip level
   3. On the anterior surface of the body

   a. 1 and 2
   b. 1 and 3
   c. 2 and 3
   d. 1, 2, and 3

10. Which of the following is(are) classified as (a) controlled area(s)?

   a. radiographic room
   b. hallway
   c. unattended elevators
   d. waiting room

11. Secondary barriers serve to shield for _____ radiation.

   1. Leakage
   2. Scatter
   3. Direct

   a. 1 and 2
   b. 1 and 3
   c. 2 and 3
   d. 1, 2, and 3

12. The Bucky slot cover provides protection for the

   a. radiographer and radiologist at the gonadal level
   b. radiographer and radiologist at the thyroid and throat level
   c. patient at the gonadal level
   d. patient at the thyroid and throat level

13. A pregnant radiographer must be issued a second personnel monitor to be worn

   a. at the collar
   b. at waist level
   c. on the wrist
   d. as a ring badge

14. For stationary x-ray units, the exposure switch must be

   a. attached to a 180-cm cord
   b. a deadman type
   c. fixed behind a protective barrier
   d. set to automatically shut off after 5 minutes

15. In order to meet linearity standards, mA stations are allowed a maximum variation of

   a. 2%
   b. 5%
   c. 10%
   d. 20%

16. The most commonly used crystal in a thermoluminescent dosimeter, which "stores" the exposure for later reading, is

   a. calcium tungstate
   b. lithium fluoride
   c. cesium iodide
   d. aluminum oxide

17. When planning protection for a diagnostic x-ray installation, the workload (w) is usually stated in

   a. R-mA/wk
   b. mA-min/week
   c. heat units (HU)/wk
   d. kV-mA min/wk

18. Protective lead barriers must extend _____ up from the floor.

   a. 5 ft
   b. 7 ft
   c. 10 ft
   d. always to ceiling height

19. The x-ray tube housing must limit leakage radiation to less than _____ mR/h at 1 m.

   a. 50
   b. 100
   c. 250
   d. 500

20. The personnel monitoring device that allows the worker to read his or her dose at the end of each workday is the

   a. film badge
   b. TLD
   c. OSL
   d. pocket dosimeter

21. Which of the following will NOT provide radiation protection for the radiographer?

    a. fluoroscopy Pb curtain
    b. film badge
    c. primary barrier
    d. Bucky slot cover

22. The wall upon which the vertical Bucky is mounted must contain

    a. 2.5 mm Al equivalent
    b. 1/32 in Pb equivalent
    c. 1/16 in Pb equivalent
    d. 0.5 mm Pb equivalent

23. A cumulative timing device runs during the x-ray exposure and sounds an audible alarm or temporarily interrupts the exposure after the fluoroscope has been activated for

    a. 30 seconds
    b. 2 minutes
    c. 5 minutes
    d. 10 minutes

24. The most sensitive type of personnel monitoring devices available because of their ability to detect exposures as low as 1 mrad is

    a. film badges
    b. thermoluminescent dosimeters
    c. optically stimulated luminescent devices
    d. monthly blood tests

25. The smallest practical dose that a standard film badge can measure is approximately

    a. 1.0 mrem (0.01 mSv)
    b. 10 mrem (0.1 mSv)
    c. 25 mrem (0.25 mSv)
    d. 100 mrem (1 mSv)

26. Which of the following is NOT a basic component of a film badge?

    a. silver halide emulsion
    b. copper filters
    c. cadmium filters
    d. self-reading meter

27. A radiographic unit is operated daily above 70 kVp. How much filtration is required to operate this machine?

    a. 2.5 mm Cd/equiv.
    b. 2.5 mm Al/equiv.
    c. 2.5 mm Pb/equiv.
    d. 2.5 mm Cu/equiv.

28. The maximum dose rate for a fixed fluoroscopy unit must be less than

    a. 100 mR/h
    b. 1 R/min
    c. 5 mR/h
    d. 10 R/min

29. Primary barriers protect against

    a. secondary radiation
    b. primary radiation
    c. leakage radiation
    d. scatter radiation

30. What is the minimum source to tabletop distance allowed for stationary fluoroscopic equipment?

    a. 12 in (30 cm)
    b. 15 in (38 cm)
    c. 40 in (100 cm)
    d. 72 in (180 cm)

Image Labeling

1. Indicate the radiation protection accuracy measurement standard that must be met for each of the labeled x-ray unit components shown.

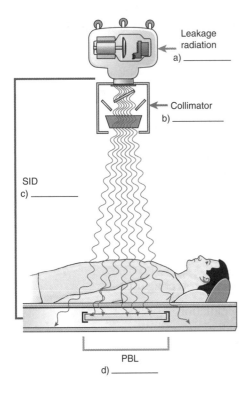

2. Fill in each lettered blank with the dose a radiographer would receive at each distance indicated with and without a lead fluoroscopic curtain in place.

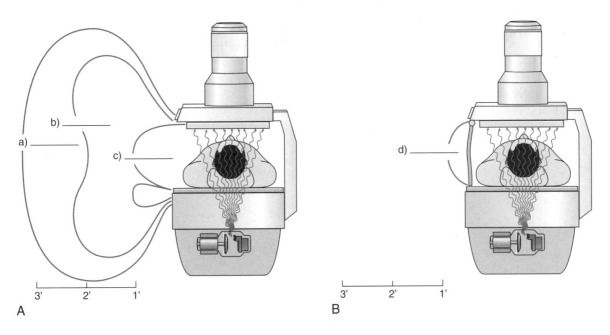

3. For each lettered item, label the type of radiation being emitted and identify whether it is considered primary or secondary radiation.

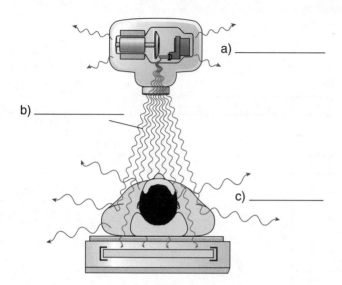

a) _____

b) _____

c) _____

Crossword Puzzle

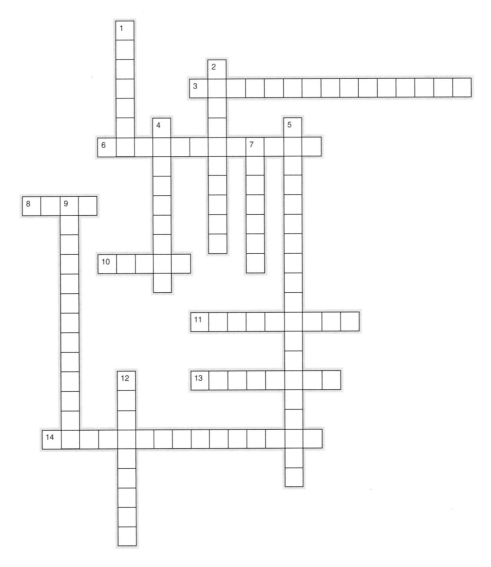

Across

3. Type of crystal used in a TLD personnel monitoring device
6. Areas where the general public can be found; includes waiting rooms and hallways
8. Most common material used in the construction of radiation protection barriers
10. Type of light used to stimulate the emission of an OSL crystal
11. The longest period of time a personnel monitor can be worn; every 3 months
13. Measured in mA-min/wk
14. Standard that states that the same technique setting should provide the same radiation intensity ±5%

Down

1. Type of exposure switch required on fluoroscopic units
2. Must be at least 2.5 mm Al equivalent for tubes operating above 70 kVp
4. General term for any dose-measuring device
5. Gas-filled survey meter
7. Type of unwanted radiation from the tube housing
9. Radiosensitive crystal used in an OSL personnel monitor
12. Type of barrier that must be 1/32 in thick

21

Minimizing Patient Exposure and Personnel Exposure

1. The radiation exposure to the technologist and radiologist can be decreased by reducing the

   a. time
   b. distance
   c. shielding
   d. monitor badge

2. Increasing the distance from the patient will cause which of the following?

   a. increase the scattered radiation reaching the staff
   b. decrease the time of radiation exposure
   c. decrease the scattered radiation reaching the staff
   d. none of the above

3. Which of the following is the source of scattered radiation during a fluoroscopy procedure?

   a. the operator
   b. the patient
   c. the image intensifier
   d. the table

4. What percent of radiation do lead aprons attenuate?

   a. 10%
   b. 50%
   c. 80%
   d. 99%

5. Which of the following technical factors can reduce radiation dose to the patient?

   a. low mAs and long time
   b. high kVp and low mAs
   c. low kVp and high mAs
   d. high kVp and high mAs

6. Lead aprons, when not in use, should be

   a. tossed in a heap
   b. placed on hanging racks
   c. folded twice and put away
   d. stuffed in a container

7. The annual effective dose limit for an occupationally exposed radiation worker is

   a. 5 mSv (0.5 rems)
   b. 50 mSv (5 rems)
   c. 1 mSv (0.1 rem)
   d. 10 mSv (1 rem)

8. The cumulative effective dose limit for a 25-year-old radiographer is

   a. 25 mSv
   b. 50 mSV
   c. 100 mSv
   d. 250 mSv

9. Lead aprons and other protective apparel should be inspected for cracks by

   1. Visual inspection
   2. Using a radiation dosimeter
   3. Using fluoroscopy

   a. 1 and 2
   b. 1 and 3
   c. 2 and 3
   d. 1, 2, and 3

10. The technologist is

    a. allowed to hold a patient during an exposure when the patient is in danger of falling
    b. allowed to hold a patient during an exposure when the patient is a baby
    c. allowed to hold a patient during an exposure when the patient is in pain
    d. never allowed to hold a patient during an exposure

11. The type of gonadal shielding that is suspended from the collimator is a

    a. flat contact shield
    b. lead apron
    c. shadow shield
    d. lead strip

12. The principle that states that patient and personnel exposure should be reduced as much as possible is often referred to as

    a. LET
    b. RBE
    c. NCRP
    d. ALARA

13. Occupationally exposed workers must wear a personnel monitor if _____ of the annual dose equivalent limit could be received.

    a. 1/10
    b. ¼
    c. ½
    d. 100%

14. The monthly effective dose limit for a declared pregnant technologist is

    a. 0.5 mSv
    b. 5.0 mSv
    c. 50 mSv
    d. 500 mSv

15. Lead aprons must have a minimum thickness of _____ when used for procedures with peak beam energies greater than 100 kVp.

    a. 2.5 mm Al
    b. 0.25 mm Pb
    c. 0.5 mm Al
    d. 0.5 mm Pb

16. The longest interval that a personnel monitor should be worn is

    a. 1 week
    b. 1 month
    c. 3 months
    d. 1 year

17. Which of the following statements best describes effective dose?

    a. the lethal dose to humans if received in one whole body exposure
    b. the dose received by the patient at the skin level
    c. the dose that accounts for biologic harm as a result of the body part that is exposed and the type of radiation used
    d. the dose of any exam as compared to a chest x-ray

18. According to the inverse square law, if a technologist doubles the distance he or she is standing from the radiation source, his or her dose will

    a. decrease to ½
    b. decrease to ¼
    c. increase two times
    d. increase four times

19. Compared to the primary beam, scatter radiation is _____.

    a. 100 times more intense
    b. 100 times less intense
    c. 1,000 times more intense
    d. 1,000 times less intense

20. Who would be the best individual to help hold a patient who is unsteady on her feet during an x-ray exposure?

    a. the patient's husband
    b. the technologist
    c. the radiologist
    d. the patient's pregnant daughter

21. The general public's effective dose limit is approximately _____ of the occupationally exposed workers.

    a. 1/100
    b. 1/10
    c. ¼
    d. ½

22. Which of the following radiations has the lowest radiation weighting factor?

    a. x-rays
    b. neutrons
    c. protons
    d. alpha

23. If the technique used for an x-ray exposure is changed from 20 to 40 mAs, the patient dose will

    a. increase two times
    b. decrease two times
    c. remain unchanged
    d. change only if kVp is changed, also

24. To calculate the effective dose received by a specific organ, the absorbed dose value is

    a. added to the tissue weighting factor
    b. multiplied by the tissue weighting factor
    c. subtracted from the tissue weighting factor
    d. divided by the tissue weighting factor

25. Which of the following radiographic examinations would cause the highest entrance skin exposure?

    a. pediatric chest x-ray
    b. PA adult chest x-ray
    c. a finger exam
    d. a lumbar spine exam

26. Which of the following actions would limit the radiation exposure to the radiologist and the technologist during fluoroscopy?

    1. Use of intermittent fluoro
    2. Pulsed fluoroscopy
    3. Continuous exposure fluoro

    a. 1 and 2
    b. 1 and 3
    c. 2 and 3
    d. 1, 2, and 3

27. The second fetal personnel monitor issued to a declared pregnant worker should be worn

    a. at the collar level
    b. as a ring badge
    c. at waist level
    d. directly over the fetus

28. Based on the tissue weighting factors, which organ is the most radiosensitive?

    a. gonads
    b. thyroid
    c. colon
    d. skin

29. The purpose of "The Ten Day Rule" is to

    a. prohibit all x-ray examinations on women of childbearing age until 10 days after menses to protect an unsuspected fetus
    b. ensure that childbearing women do not have any abdominal or pelvic examinations during the menstrual period
    c. limit abdominal and pelvic region examinations to the first 10 days of the menstrual cycle to protect an unsuspected fetus
    d. allow women of childbearing age up to 10 days to schedule all abdomen/pelvic x-ray examination

30. During a fluoroscopic examination, which of the following would be the BEST place for the radiographer to stand in order to minimize his or her exposure?

    a. as close as possible to the examining table
    b. as far away as practical from the examining table
    c. at the patient's head
    d. facing away from the fluoro tower and image intensifier

Image Labeling

1. Complete the table by listing the radiation weighting factor assigned to each type of radiation.

Type and Energy Range	Radiation Weighting Factor (Wr)
X and gamma rays, electrons	
Neutrons, energy	
<10 keV	
10–100 keV	
>100 keV to 2 MeV	
>29 MeV	
Protons	
Alpha particles	

2. Complete the table by identifying the dose equivalent limit set for each radiation worker factor listed.

Occupational Exposures	Dose Limit Values
Effective dose limits a. Annual b. Cumulative	
Equivalent annual dose limits for tissues and organs a. Lens of eye b. Skin, hands, and feet	
Public exposure (annual) Effective dose limit a. Continuous or frequent exposure b. Infrequent exposure	
Equivalent dose limits for tissues and organs a. Lens of eye b. Skin, hands, and feet	
Embryo/fetus exposures a. Total equivalent dose limit b. Monthly equivalent dose limit	
Education and training exposures (annual) Effective dose limit	
Equivalent dose limits for tissues and organs a. Lens of eye b. Skin, hands, and feet	

3. Identify the different exposure levels to the radiographer when distance is changed.

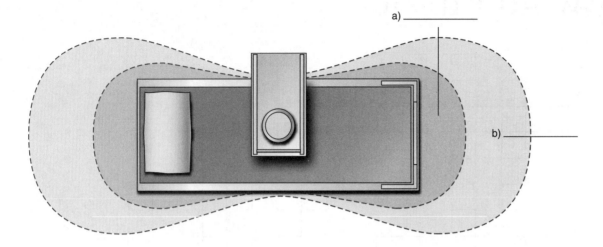

a) _____

b) _____

Crossword Puzzle

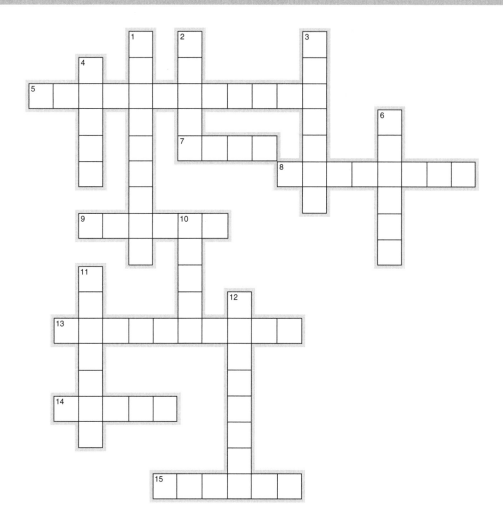

Across

5. SI unit used to measure effective dose
7. One of the three cardinal rules of radiation protection; measures in seconds and minutes
8. The frequency that lead aprons are inspected for cracks
9. The rule that states that all elective abdominal radiographs on women of childbearing age should be postponed until this period
13. The dose limit calculated using the formula: age × 10 mSv
14. The designated period of time that it is allowable for a technologist to stand in the primary beam
15. The relationship between mAs and patient dose

Down

1. One of the three cardinal principles of radiation protection; involves using a barrier
2. The level where the second fetal badge should be worn
3. The primary source of scatter and occupational dose for the radiographer
4. The type of radiation that has the highest radiation weighting factor
6. Type of gonadal shield that is suspended from the collimator
10. As low as reasonably achievable
11. Each repeat exposure does this to patient dose
12. One of the three cardinal principles of radiation protection; best practice is to keep this as great as possible

PART VI

Patient Care

22

Medical and Professional Ethics

1. Which of the following guarantees that the
   health information of the patient remains
   private?

   a. autonomy
   b. ASRT
   c. HIPAA
   d. charting

2. Which principle of the Code of Ethics states that
   the Radiologic Technologist provides services to
   patients without discrimination?

   a. 1
   b. 2
   c. 3
   d. 4

3. The unlawful touching of a person without his
   or her consent in an injurious way is known as

   a. battery
   b. assault
   c. slander
   d. invasion of privacy

4. When the patient's information is maliciously
   spread in a verbal format, this is known as

   a. libel
   b. battery
   c. assault
   d. slander

5. Which of the following are hallmarks of a
   profession?

   1. Sets practice standards
   2. Determines appropriate education levels
   3. Advances knowledge through research

   a. 1 and 2
   b. 1 and 3
   c. 2 and 3
   d. 1, 2, and 3

6. Which Code of Ethics principle deals with
   continuing education for the radiographer?

   a. 3
   b. 6
   c. 8
   d. 10

7. Professional ethics are defined as/by

   a. each technologist's moral compass
   b. the patient's expectations
   c. a set of moral principles that govern an
      individual's course of action
   d. the determination of right and wrong based on
      past experiences

8. The Code of Ethics that has the radiographer exercise care, discretion, and judgment to the patient is found in

   a. Principle 5
   b. Principle 6
   c. Principle 7
   d. Principle 8

9. If a technologist routinely fails to collimate, shield patients, and use appropriate technical factors, he or she has failed to observe which Principle from the Code of Ethics?

   a. Principle 5
   b. Principle 6
   c. Principle 7
   d. Principle 8

10. When a patient is administered contrast, a radiographer should chart the contrast used, the time of the procedure, and any

    a. position that the patient is in
    b. reaction that the patient experienced
    c. technical factors that were used
    d. none of the above

11. The ethical principle that deals with truthfulness is

    a. beneficence
    b. justice
    c. veracity
    d. fidelity

12. Which of the following is NOT considered a patient right?

    a. the right to receive considerate care
    b. the right to confidentiality
    c. the right to receive the results of an examination
    d. the right to fair compensation

13. A crime against a person or property is called a(n)

    a. tort
    b. felony
    c. misdemeanor
    d. infraction

14. The inappropriate use of restraints during a radiographic examination could result in an intentional tort of

    a. false imprisonment
    b. libel
    c. battery
    d. negligence

15. When can medical information be released to a third party such as an employer or other medical facilities?

    a. when a physician deems it is in the best interest of the patient
    b. when a relative requests the information for the patient
    c. when the patient has given express written consent for this action
    d. never

16. If a patient is not appropriately covered during a radiographic examination, the radiographer risks being charged with

    a. negligence
    b. invasion of privacy
    c. assault
    d. slander

17. Which of the following is NOT a condition that must exist to establish a claim of malpractice?

    a. a duty to provide reasonable care to the patient existed
    b. the patient suffered a loss or injury
    c. the defendant is the party responsible for the loss or injury
    d. the loss must be tied to damage from radiation exposure

18. Entries in a patient chart or medical record should be

    a. objective
    b. subjective
    c. pejorative
    d. perfunctory

19. Which of the following are relevant items to obtain and document as part of the patient's history prior to commencing a radiographic examination?

    1. Reason for the exam
    2. Possibility of pregnancy
    3. Level of patient's education

    a. 1 and 2
    b. 1 and 3
    c. 2 and 3
    d. 1, 2, and 3

20. Which of the following actions is NOT within a radiographer's scope of practice?

    a. identifying a patient using information provided by the patient and the hospital
    b. diagnosing and interpreting the medical images he or she has obtained
    c. using diagnostic techniques for all radiographic exposures
    d. representing the profession outside one's place of employment

21. Which agency is in charge of enforcing the Rules of Ethics for Radiologic Technologists?

    a. ARRT
    b. ASRT
    c. HIPAA
    d. ISRRT

22. A radiographer may be found guilty of a tort if which of the following type of behavior is demonstrated?

    1. Talking about a patient's exam with the patient's and technologist's mutual friend
    2. Performing an exam on a patient who has refused the exam
    3. Performing an exam under orders from the ER physician rather than the patient's primary care physician

    a. 1 and 2
    b. 1 and 3
    c. 2 and 3
    d. 1, 2, and 3

23. Allowing patients to make their own decisions about their medical care aligns with the ethical principle of

    a. autonomy
    b. beneficence
    c. fidelity
    d. justice

24. A patient sustains an injury from a fall after being briefly left unattended. In this case, the technologist could be held liable for

    a. libel
    b. malpractice
    c. negligence
    d. fidelity

25. Which organization is responsible for drafting and maintaining the Patient's Bill of Rights?

    a. AHA
    b. ASRT
    c. AFL-CIO
    d. FDA

26. When documenting patient information on paper, which of the following is not an acceptable practice?

    a. notations must be in ink
    b. the date and signature of the person making the notation should be included
    c. personal shorthand and abbreviations may be used
    d. direct observations of patient behavior during an exam may be included

27. Which actions help to ensure the confidentiality of electronic medical records?

    1. Logging off after entering patient data
    2. Using universal passwords for the department
    3. Using barcodes for patient and/or technologist identification

    a. 1 and 2
    b. 1 and 3
    c. 2 and 3
    d. 1, 2, and 3

28. When an entry in a medical record needs to be corrected, the technologist should

    a. use whiteout and write over the change
    b. tape an extra sheet of paper beside the change, explaining the error
    c. completely cover the error with a black ink pen, initial it, and add the corrected information underneath
    d. draw a line through the error, add the correct information, and initial and date the change

29. Which type of crime is usually punishable by imprisonment?

    a. torts
    b. felonies
    c. misdemeanors
    d. nonmaleficence

30. If corporate negligence is found to have occurred, which party will be held liable for the damages?

    a. the technologist
    b. the radiologist
    c. the hospital
    d. the technologist with partial cause resting with the patient

Crossword Puzzle

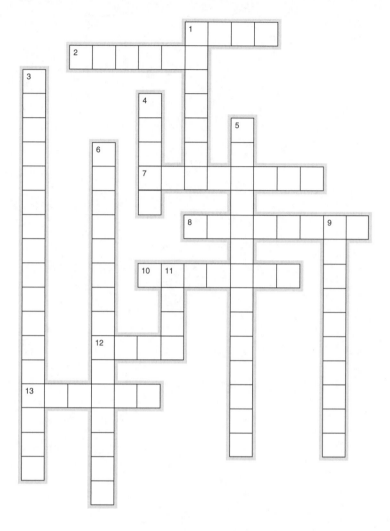

Across

1. The acronym for the agency that oversees certification and registration of technologists in the United States
2. A set of moral principles that govern an individual's course of action
7. The ethical principle that represents self-determination
8. The process of placing notes, patient history, diagnoses, and other medical information in a patient's medical record
10. An intentional tort that can result if a radiographer proceeds with an exam despite the patient's refusal
12. The type of law that involves personal injury or damage to property; handled in civil courts
13. A set of personal behaviors based on lessons of right and wrong learned at an early age

Down

1. An intentional tort; the unlawful threat of touching a person in an injurious way
3. Tort that would result if a patient was restrained against his or her will
4. Health Insurance Portability and Accountability Act
5. The duty or obligation to prevent harm
6. The radiographer has the duty to maintain the patient's _____ at all times; holding patient information in trust
9. The neglect or omission of reasonable care or caution
11. Acronym for the professional organization of the radiologic sciences in the United States

23

Patient Care, Medications, Vital Signs, and Body Mechanics

1. Needle size is measured using _____ sizes.

   a. French
   b. length
   c. gauge
   d. syringe

2. Which of the following has different tube lengths to connect the needle to a syringe?

   a. winged needle or butterfly needle
   b. angiocath needle
   c. straight needle
   d. curved needle

3. Which of the following solutions can be used to clean the injection site prior to venipuncture?

   a. alcohol
   b. soap and water
   c. bleach
   d. ionic benzoic acid

4. When inserting a needle into a vein, the bore on the bevel side should be

   a. up
   b. down
   c. sideways
   d. none of the above

5. Plastic syringes are used because they can be

   a. sterilized and reused
   b. disposed of
   c. seen better
   d. sent home with the patient

6. Which blood tests are used prior to any injection of contrast media?

   1. Glucose
   2. BUN
   3. Creatinine

   a. 1 and 2
   b. 1 and 3
   c. 2 and 3
   d. 1, 2, and 3

7. Any iodine-containing contrast can cause a reaction known as

   a. hemostasis
   b. anaphylaxis
   c. hypertension
   d. bradypnea

8. Which device is used to take blood pressure measurements?

   a. spectrometer
   b. thermometer
   c. Luer-lock syringe
   d. sphygmomanometer

9. Normal blood pressure for an adult is considered to be

   a. 100/50
   b. 119/79
   c. 180/120
   d. 140/100

10. The normal pulse rate for a resting adult is

    a. 30 to 50 beats/min
    b. 60 to 100 beats/min
    c. 90 to 130 beats/min
    d. 100 to 150 beats/min

11. When the pulse rate is <60 beats/min, this is known as

    a. bradycardia
    b. tachycardia
    c. dyscardia
    d. shock

12. The normal respiration rate for an adult at rest is _____ breaths/min.

    a. 12 to 20
    b. 18 to 26
    c. 20 to 30
    d. 25 to 36

13. The normal oral body temperature for an adult is

    a. 68.5°F
    b. 72.6°F
    c. 98.6°F
    d. 101°F

14. The axillary and rectal temperatures vary by _____ degree(s) from the normal oral temperature.

    a. 1
    b. 3
    c. 5
    d. 10

15. The body parts that are most likely to be injured if poor body mechanics is used during patient transfer maneuvers is the

    a. forearms and humerus
    b. lower legs and femur
    c. back and lumbar spine
    d. neck and cervical spine

16. Which of the following sites could be used to determine a patient's pulse?

    a. carotid artery
    b. femoral artery
    c. radial artery
    d. all of the above

17. All of the vital signs include

    a. temperature, pulse, and respiration
    b. temperature, pulse, respiration, and blood pressure
    c. temperature, pulse, and blood pressure
    d. pulse, heart rate, and blood count

18. If a patient does not need to be transported on a cart for a chest examination, he or she may be transported using a

    a. mobile radiographic unit
    b. wheelchair
    c. slide board
    d. hydraulic lift

19. Possible adverse reactions to an intravenously injected iodinated contrast media include

    a. urticaria
    b. dyspnea
    c. hypotension
    d. all of the above

20. During an intravenous contrast exam, the technologist notes that infiltration and extravasation have occurred. The appropriate actions to be taken by the technologist include

    a. flushing the tubing with a sterile sodium chloride solution
    b. administering oxygen and monitoring the patient's vital signs
    c. applying cold compresses and discontinuing the injection
    d. nothing; these are only mild and transitory reactions to the contrast media

21. The first action a technologist should take when transferring an appropriately identified patient from bed to wheelchair is

    a. positioning the wheelchair parallel to the bed
    b. locking the wheels
    c. placing the good leg down first
    d. placing the patient in a semi-Fowler/high Fowler position

22. Which of the following needle or angiocath gauge size would be the most appropriate for IV contrast administration?

    a. 26
    b. 18
    c. 10
    d. 1

23. Prior to beginning venipuncture, the technologist should

    a. wash his or her hands
    b. suit up in a surgical gown and gloves
    c. tape the butterfly needle in place
    d. check that hemostasis has occurred

24. After the administration of an iodinated contrast medium, how long should the patient be monitored for any adverse reactions?

    a. for the duration of the injection only
    b. 1 minute
    c. 10 minutes
    d. 20 minutes

25. The type of iodinated contrast medium that is less likely to cause adverse reactions is

    a. ionic
    b. nonionic
    c. benzoic
    d. creatinine

26. Which is the preferred injection site for most radiographic contrast administration exams?

    a. radial artery
    b. pulmonary vein
    c. apical pulse point
    d. antecubital vein

27. Which of the following is not a principle of good body mechanics?

    a. providing a wide base of support
    b. bending your knees when lifting
    c. twisting, rather than pivoting
    d. rolling or pulling a heavy object

28. If a technologist is not able to transfer a patient safely, he or she should

    a. use the hydraulic lift
    b. seek assistance from another health care professional
    c. use a slide board and draw sheet simultaneously
    d. notify the physician that the exam is being canceled

29. The minimum number of individuals needed to safely complete a draw sheet patient transfer is

    a. 1
    b. 2
    c. 4
    d. 5

30. In order for venipuncture to be successful,

    a. the tourniquet must be applied 3 inches above the carotid artery
    b. the vein must curve along the axis of the arm
    c. the vein must be at least two times the diameter of the needle
    d. the arm should be raised for a few seconds first to allow the blood to travel back to the heart

Image Labeling

1. Label the relevant components of a venipuncture procedure.

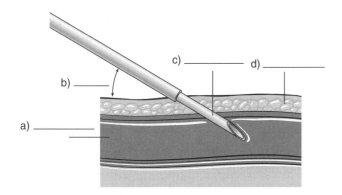

2. Identify the parts of the syringe shown.

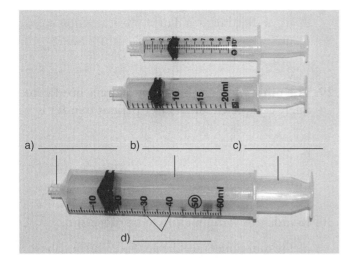

3. Complete the lettered components of the sphygmomanometer.

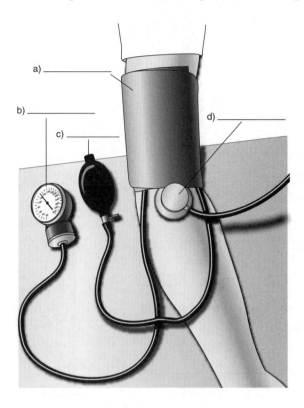

4. Label the common human pulse points as shown on the diagram.

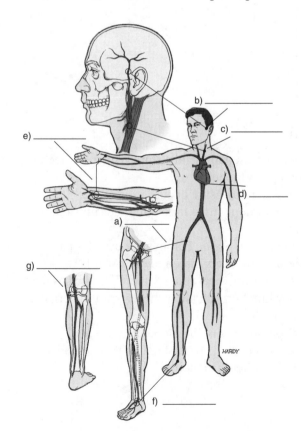

Crossword Puzzle

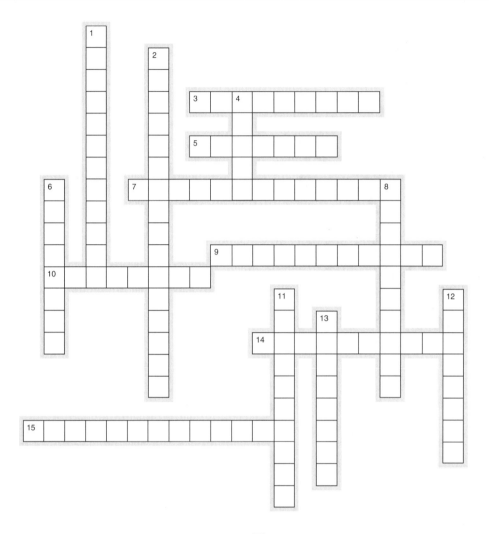

Across

3. Needle with a flexible catheter
5. Fits inside the syringe; used to push the medication out of the syringe
7. Principles used to ensure proper alignment, balance, and movement in order to prevent worker injuries
9. Condition that exists when an adult has pulse rates over 100 beats/min
10. Type of syringe used with straight steel needles; provides a secure connection
14. Condition where bleeding has discontinued; needs to be established before dismissing a patient after an IV procedure
15. Complication of venipuncture when contrast media has leaked out of the vessel

Down

1. Procedure used to establish an IV site for injection
2. Blood pressure cuff
4. Unit used to measure needle sizes
6. Vein commonly used for contrast administration in radiology
8. Rigid sheet of plastic that may be used for patient transfer maneuvers in lieu of draw sheets
11. A normal value between 0.8 and 1.3 indicates that kidney function will allow the contrast material to be cleared
12. The top number of the blood pressure reading
13. Type of iodinated contrast media that is less likely to cause patient reactions

Laboratory Experiments

Electric and Magnetic Fields

Name: _____   Date: _____

Electrostatics is the study of stationary or resting electric charges. An electric field exists around all electric charges. An English scientist, Michael Faraday (1791–1867), introduced the concept of using lines of force as an aid in visualizing the magnitude and direction of an electric field. Similarly, the magnetic force per unit pole is called the magnetic field. In this case, the field is mapped out by using the poles of magnets. The purpose of this activity is to allow the student to visualize and map both electric and magnetic fields and compare their similarities and differences.

Objectives:

Upon completion of this lab, the student will be able to:

1. Draw the electric field surrounding both positive and negative charges.
2. Visualize and draw the magnetic field surrounding magnets.
3. Apply the laws of electrostatic and magnetic fields to his or her drawing.
4. Compare and contrast the similarities and differences in electric and magnetic fields and their respective laws of interaction.

Part I: Electrostatic Fields

Draw the electric fields for each charge configuration below, indicating the lines of force, and/or their interactions as applicable. After you have completed your sketches, answer the questions.

a. The electric field of a single point charge

+

b. The electric field of two like point charges

+   +

c. The electric field of two unlike point charges

+   −

1. What are the main differences between items B and C? What law of electrostatics is illustrated in both of these situations?

_____

_____

_____

2. In situation C, if the force represented at the current distance is equal to 3 N, what would be the new force if the distance between the charges was increased? Complete the sentence below with your answer.

   If the distances between the charges are increased, then the force of the _____ (attraction/repulsion) will be _____ (increased/decreased).
   a. Whose law is being applied here?

_____

_____

_____

Part II: Magnetic Fields

Materials:

1. Two bar magnets
2. Iron filings
3. Paper

Procedure:

1. Cover the bar magnets with a sheet of paper in the following configurations:
   a. A single bar magnet.
   b. Two bar magnets with the north and south poles next to each other with approximately 5 cm separating each magnetic pole.
   c. Two bar magnets with the south and south poles next to each other with approximately 5 cm apart separating each magnetic pole.

2. Sprinkle an ample amount of iron filings on top of the paper in order to obtain a visible pattern of the magnetic field.

3. Sketch the observed magnetic field patterns for each configuration, rendering the field lines as close to actual size as possible.

4. After the patterns have been sketched, collect the iron filings using your paper as a "funnel," and return them to the container (recycling them for someone else's use).

5. Complete your sketches by indicating the direction of the magnetic field lines. Attach your drawings to this lab report, and answer the following questions.

Analysis:

1. Look at your drawing for the single bar magnet. What happens to the distance between the field lines as the distance increases from the magnet?

_____

_____

_____

2. Evaluate the difference in the magnetic fields for configurations b and c. What law of magnetism is being illustrated?

_____

_____

_____

3. If the magnets in configuration b were moved farther apart, what would happen to the force of attraction/repulsion? Whose law would be illustrated in this case?

_____

_____

_____

4. Compare the electric and magnetic field arrangements you sketched. Describe the differences and similarities between the fields and the laws that they obey?

_____

_____

_____

5. What is the one fundamental difference between electric charges versus magnetic poles?

_____

_____

_____

Faraday's Law

Name: _____ Date: _____`

Michael Faraday is credited with discovering electromagnetic induction: When a wire moves or magnetic field changes so that the flux (field) lines are cut by the wire, an EMF will be induced in the wire. Electromagnetic induction is an important fundamental principle, because it is the basis for the operation of various components in the x-ray tube and circuit.

Faraday's law explains that the induced voltage (EMF) in a coil is proportional to the product of the number of loops and the rate at which the magnetic field changes within the loops. This lab provides students with the opportunity to test various aspects of Faraday's law and observe the effects of electromagnetic induction.

Objectives:

Upon the completion of this lab, the student will be able to:

1. Describe the conditions that must be present in order for electromagnetic induction to occur.
2. Demonstrate and describe the following aspects of Faraday's law:
   a. Demonstrate and describe the type of motion necessary to induce voltage using a conductor and a magnet.
   b. Determine what effects the number of loops and motion have on the amount of voltage induced.

Materials:

1. Galvanometer
2. Bar magnet
3. Long solenoid
4. Short solenoid
5. Black and red connecting wires

Procedure:

1. Connect the positive and negative ends of the galvanometer to the positive and negative ends of the long solenoid. When connected correctly, the galvanometer should register current when the magnet is moved inside the galvanometer. Follow the instructions and answer the questions as indicated.

Data and Analysis:

1. Insert the bar magnet into the coil. What happened to the needle/display? What does the galvanometer register?

   _____

   _____

   _____

2. Leave the magnet stationary inside the coil. What does the galvanometer read now?

   _____

   _____

   _____

3. Slide the magnet back and forth repeatedly inside the coil. Document the galvanometer results.

   _____

   _____

   _____

4. Move the magnet up and down repeatedly inside the coil. Record the galvanometer results.

   _____

   _____

   _____

5. Hold the magnet stationary. Rapidly move the coil back and forth around the magnet. Record the galvanometer readings.

   _____

   _____

   _____

6. Connect the short solenoid coil to the galvanometer using the same connections outlined in the "Procedure" section. Repeat Step 3. Record the new galvanometer readings. How does this value compare with the longer solenoid?

_____

_____

_____

7. Based on your results above, what conditions must exist in order to produce voltage and current according to Faraday's law? (List all that apply.)

_____

_____

_____

Effect of Technical Factors on X-ray Beam Intensity and Exposure Indicator Numbers

Name: _____   Date: _____

The primary technical factors that a technologist uses to ensure a proper exposure and appearance of the image are mA, time, and kVp. Each of these factors can be changed independently, and each has an effect on the total exposure received by the patient and the image receptor. As a result, each affects the Exposure Indicator Number of the digital imaging system being used. It is essential that a technologist understands the effect that each technique change has on the x-ray beam's quantity and the subsequent effect this has on the Exposure Indicator Number. Understanding this relationship provides the technologist with the ability to apply the proper technique rules if corrective factors are needed in the case of an improperly exposed image.

Objectives:

Upon completion of this lab, the student will be able to:

1. Independently set kVp, time, and mA.
2. Properly use an ionization chamber or R-meter to measure x-ray machine output.
3. Evaluate the effect of technique changes on radiographic images.
4. Evaluate the effect of technique changes on Exposure Indicator Numbers.
5. Synthesize the relationships between the technique changes and the visual image changes and the Exposure number changes.

Materials:

1. Energized radiographic unit
2. R-meter or ionization chamber
3. Computed radiographic unit or DR unit
4. Knee phantom
5. Lead markers to number each exposure

Procedure:

1. Place the knee phantom in an AP position and expose using a Bucky technique that will provide an acceptable Exposure Indicator Number. Suggested techniques are below but may need to be adjusted for the x-ray unit and CR unit being used.

Exposure no. 1: 100 mA	150 ms	65 kVp (**Base technique**)
Exposure no. 2: **200 mA**	150 ms	65kVp
Exposure no. 3: 100 mA	**300 ms**	65 kVp
Exposure no. 4: 100 mA	150 ms	**75 kVp**

2. Number each exposure of the knee, and change the technique factors relative to the suggested techniques shown: (Be sure to maintain the same collimation throughout.)

   a. For Exposure no. 2, double the mA from the base technique.
   b. For Exposure no. 3, double the time from the base technique.
   c. For Exposure no. 4, increase the kVp by 15% (~10 KVp).

3. Evaluate each image and record the Exposure Indicator Number in the Data Table provided.

4. Repeat Exposures 1 to 4, this time only placing the R-meter in the beam. Record each reading in the Data Table, resetting the meter after each exposure.

5. Analyze the results by answering the questions provided.

Data:

Exposure No.	Technique		Image Density/Brightness	Exposure Indicator Number	X-ray Intensity (mR)
	kVp	mAs			
1					
2					
3					
4					

Analysis:

1. **Visually evaluate the radiographic images. Which exposure provided (a) diagnostic image(s)? List them here:**

   a. What change in density (or brightness) was noted in the images with each technique change made? Explain why the image change occurred (or did not occur).

   _____

   _____

   _____

2. **Evaluate the Exposure Indicator Numbers for each exposure. Were all of the exposure numbers in the acceptable range for the unit being used? List the exposures which were and were not in the acceptable range.**

    a. As each technique change was made, did the Exposure Number go up or down in value?

    _____

    _____

    _____

    b. Based on your answer to 2a and the direction of the technique change made, is this system's Exposure Number proportional (in the same direction) as the technique change or inverse (in the opposite direction) of the technique change?

    _____

    _____

    _____

3. **Evaluate the x-ray intensity readings for each exposure. What trend(s) do you note with each technique factor change?**

    _____

    _____

    _____

4. **Compare the Exposure Indicator Number with the mR reading obtained for each exposure. What relationship do you note between these two values for each exposure?**

    a. Based on your answer, what relationship can you make between the Exposure Indicator Number and the exposure received by the image receptor?

    _____

    _____

    _____

5. Based on your results, predict what changes would occur in the Exposure
    Indicator Number and the x-ray intensity values if each technique factor was cut to one
    half of the base technique.

    _____

    _____

    _____

6. Using your results, explain how the Exposure Indicator Number can be used to
    correct an improperly exposed digital image.

    _____

    _____

    _____

Effect of kVp on Radiographic Contrast

Name: _____   Date: _____

kVp is responsible for altering the energy, wavelength, and penetration ability of the x-beam. Changing the energy of the beam also affects the final radiograph. This lab is designed to demonstrate the effects of changing kVp on image contrast and gray scale.

Objectives:

Upon the completion of this lab, the student will be able to:

1. Accurately use a densitometer.
2. Evaluate radiographic images, accurately describing their image contrast.
3. Mathematically calculate image contrast.
4. Describe the effects of kVp on radiographic contrast.

Materials:

1. Knee or lower extremity phantom
2. Two 10 × 12 cassettes
3. Densitometer
4. Leaded markers (no. 1, no. 2)
5. Calculator

Procedure:

1. Produce two images of the knee using a Bucky grid, one on each film using the two widely varying kVps. Exposure no. 1 should be exposed at 60 to 65 kVp. Exposure no. 2 should be exposed at 90 kVp. Adjust the mAs so that density is maintained.

2. Techniques:

   Exposure no. 1 _____ kVp   _____ mAs
   Exposure no. 2 _____ kVp   _____ mAs

3. Process each film using a properly warmed-up automatic film processor.

4. Take density readings of the areas of the knee described for each exposure, placing your data in the appropriate spaces.

5. Answer and complete the analysis section questions based on your observations and data for the knee images.

Data:

Record the density readings for each AP knee image taken:

Exposure no. 1 Medial Epicondyle (Area A) _____
         Midpoint of patella (Area B) _____

Exposure no. 2 Medial Epicondyle (Area A) _____
         Midpoint of patella (Area B) _____

Analysis:

1. **Visually inspect the two knee images. Which radiograph exhibits the highest contrast?** _____

2. **Calculate the contrast on each exposure by dividing the larger density value by the smaller density value (i.e., A/B) for each exposure and record below:**

Contrast:

Exposure no. 1_____
Exposure no. 2_____

1. According to your contrast calculations, which knee radiograph has the highest contrast?

   a. Does this agree with your visual analysis? Why or why not?

   _____

   _____

2. Based on your results, what effect does increasing kVp have on contrast?

   _____

   _____

3. Do your results agree with the expected results? If not, what reason(s) might explain this?

   _____

   _____

Field Size: Effects on Density and Contrast

Name: _____   Date: _____

Field size is an important contributor to diagnostic quality and patient dose. Collimation restricts the total number of the patient's atoms interacting with the primary beam, automatically reducing patient dose. In turn, fewer atoms will produce Compton interactions, decreasing scatter radiation and image fog. This lab provides students with the opportunity to evaluate the effects that large and small field sizes have on density and contrast.

Objectives:

Upon completion of this lab, the student will be able to:

1. Analyze changes in image density between a large and small field size.
2. Analyze changes in image contrast between a large and small field size.
3. Use a densitometer and calculations to mathematically analyze the differences between density and contrast for two images with different field sizes.
4. Outline reasons for collimating in terms of image quality and patient dose.

Materials:

1. Energized x-ray unit
2. Abdomen phantom
3. 14 × 17 cassette (or field size) and an 8 × 10-in cassette (or field size)
4. Densitometer

Procedure:

1. Place the abdomen in a lateral position directly on the 14 × 17-in image receptor on the tabletop (do not use a grid).
2. Center on the lumbar spine and open the collimator to its full 17 × 17 in size.
3. Expose using the suggested technique (20 mAs at 80 kVp) or another technique provided by your instructor.
4. Process the image.
5. For Exposure no. 2, use an 8 × 10-in image receptor; collimate to a 5 × 5 in field size if possible, keeping the same centering and technique as Exposure no. 1.
6. Process the image.

7. On both images, select and circle two homogenous densities: one in the soft tissue/intervertebral joint space (Area A) and the second one in an area of bony anatomy (Area B).
8. Using a densitometer, complete the Data Table for Area A and Area B.
9. To calculate contrast for each exposure, divide the Area A density by the Area B density.
10. Complete the Data Table and answer the questions as indicated.

Data:

Exposure No.	Area A Density	Area B Density	Contrast (A/B)
1			
2			

Analysis:

1. Visually compare Exposure no. 1 with Exposure no. 2. What happened to density when the field size was reduced?

   _____

   _____

   _____

2. Evaluate your densitometer readings for the Area A density for Exposure nos. 1 and 2. According to your data, which exposure has the lowest density?

   a. Does this agree with your visual analysis? Why or why not?

   _____

   _____

   _____

3. Divide Exposure no. 2's Area A density by Exposure no. 1's Area A density. Multiply this amount by 100: _____

   This represents the percentage of density remaining in Exposure no. 2 after collimating.

4. Visually analyze Exposure no. 1 and Exposure no. 2 again. Which image has the highest contrast?

_____

_____

_____

5. Refer to your Data Table. Compare the contrast values of both exposures. According to your calculations, which image has the highest contrast?

   a. Does this agree with your visual analysis? Why or why not?

   _____

   _____

   _____

6. In a brief paragraph, describe why these changes in density and contrast occur when field size is reduced.

_____

_____

_____

7. Why are smaller field sizes preferable? Address both image quality and patient dose in your answer.

_____

_____

_____

Image Receptor Effect on Density and Contrast

Name: _____   Date: _____

The image receptor is responsible for absorbing the remnant radiation that exits the patient and converting it to a visible image. This is accomplished using conventional screen/film or using digital imaging systems. The ideal image receptor provides the highest detail possible using the lowest exposure factors. Several different system speeds are available, and in order to maintain density when changing from one screen speed to another, the following conversion formula needs to be used: $mAs_2 = mAs_1 \times$ (old screen speed/new screen speed). Different image receptor systems also can affect contrast. This lab provides students with the opportunity to expose various types of image receptors and compare their effects on density and contrast.

Objectives:

Upon completion of this lab, the student will be able to:

1. Calculate the exposure factor conversions needed for different system speeds.
2. Evaluate radiographs for density and contrast.
3. Compare different image receptor systems' effects on density and contrast.

Materials:

1. Hand phantom
2. Two different screen/film combinations and one digital imaging option
3. Energized x-ray unit
4. Lead markers to number exposures
5. View boxes
6. Densitometer

Procedure:

1. Using the hand phantom, make three exposures on different image receptor systems as indicated below. For best results and easier comparison, complete your answer tables so that "Exposure no. 1" is the fastest speed system used, and "Exposure no. 3" is the slowest

speed system. (You do not have to take the exposures in this order, just complete the table this way so that the questions will be applicable.)

2. Expose the phantom by placing it directly on the image receptor using a technique provided by your instructor to obtain an image of diagnostic quality.

3. Convert the technique from the first diagnostic image using the formula in the introduction so that density is maintained for the remaining two exposures. (See the suggested conversion factors at the end of this section.)

4. Select a darker gray soft tissue area on each image (with the exception of the digital image), circle it, and label it Area A. Select a bony area, circle it on each image, and label it Area B. Take densitometer measurements of each circled area.

5. Complete the Data Tables and answer the analysis questions as indicated

SUGGESTED CONVERSION FACTORS

Screen	Relative Speed
Par	100
Hi-Plus	200
Ortho-Detail	400
CR Imaging plate	400
Ortho-Regular	800
Direct Exposure	3.3

Data:

TABLE 1 IMAGE RECEPTORS AND DENSITY

Exposure No.	IR and Imaging Speed	Total mAs Used	Area A OD	Area B OD

TABLE 2 IMAGE RECEPTORS AND CONTRAST

Exposure No.	IR and Imaging Speed	Contrast A/B*

*Divide the larger OD value by the smaller OD value.

Analysis:

1. On a view box, visually compare the overall optical densities for all of the film/screen exposures. Are there any exposures where density is inadequate and/or too great? List them here.

_____

_____

_____

2. Did the technique changes used for the different system speeds reasonably maintain density? For any images for which density was not maintained, what specific technical factor change(s) would have worked better according to your data? (HINT: Use your density readings and mAs values to help you determine this.)

_____

_____

_____

3. If this change in screens were made when going FROM Exposure no. 1 TO the last exposure (Exposure no. 3) without adjusting technique, what would happen to the resulting density?

_____

_____

_____

4. Based on your findings, what effect does image receptor speed have on density?

_____

_____

_____

5. Visually compare the contrast for all of the film exposures. Identify the system with the highest contrast and the system with the lowest contrast.

_____

_____

_____

6. Complete Data Table 2 by computing the image contrast for each exposure.

   a. Which system had the highest computed contrast?

   _____

   _____

   _____

   b. Which system had the lowest computed contrast?

   _____

   _____

   _____

7. Compare your visual findings in Question 1 to your densitometer readings in Data Table 1. Report your findings versus the expected findings. Did they agree? Why or why not?

_____

_____

_____

8. Compare your visual findings in Question 5 to your computed contrast values in Data Table 2. Report your findings versus the expected findings. Did they agree? Why or why not?

_____

_____

_____

9. What general rule can you synthesize regarding image receptor speed contrast?

_____

_____

_____

10a. Evaluate the computed radiography image in terms of density and contrast. Describe the image's density compared to the other film-based images:

_____

_____

_____

Record the Exposure Indicator Number here: _____
Is this in the optimal exposure range? _____
If not, what new technique would you recommend?

_____

_____

_____

10b. Compared to the image that you selected as the most optimal:

Is the contrast higher or lower? _____
Is the gray scale longer or shorter? _____

How does a CR-based system differ from a film-based system that would explain this difference in terms of contrast?

_____

_____

_____

Receptor Effect on Image Blur and Sharpness of Detail

Name: _____   Date: _____

As discussed in the previous lab, the image receptor is responsible for capturing the remnant radiation that exits the patient and converting it to a visible image. Both conventional screen and film or digital imaging systems can be used to accomplish this. The ideal image receptor provides the highest detail possible using the lowest exposure factors. The previous lab evaluated the effects of image receptors on density and contrast. This lab will investigate the effects of image receptors on image blur and sharpness of detail

Objectives:

Upon completion of this lab, the student will be able to:

1. Use and evaluate a line pair resolution tool.
2. Evaluate radiographs for sharpness of detail and image blur.
3. Compare different image receptor systems' effects on sharpness of detail and image blur.

Materials:

1. Hand images from the Image Receptor Lab conducted to evaluate the effects on density and contrast
2. Two different screen/film combinations and one digital imaging option
3. Energized x-ray unit
4. Line pair resolution test tool
5. Lead markers to number exposures
6. Viewboxes
7. Densitometer

Procedure:

1. Using the same techniques and image receptor systems as the Image Receptor Lab conducted for density and contrast, expose the resolution test pattern. **Place the resolution test pattern on a 1-in sponge for each exposure.**

2. Number each exposure on different image receptor systems as indicated below. For best results and easier comparison, complete your answer tables so that "Exposure no. 1" is the fastest speed system used, and your last exposure (Exposure no. 3) is the slowest speed system.

3. Evaluate your hand images for detail and image blur.

4. Complete the Data Table and answer the analysis questions as indicated.

Data:

TABLE 1 IMAGE RECEPTORS AND IMAGE BLUR

Exposure No.	IR and Imaging Speed	Resolution (lp/mm)

Analysis:

1. Visually examine the anatomy and bony trabeculae of all three exposures. Which exposure appears to have the greatest detail and which one has the least?

_____

_____

_____

2. Refer to the Data Table. Which image receptor resolved the greatest number of line pairs per millimeter and which one the least?

   a. Does this agree with your visual observations?

   _____

   _____

3. Why does this effect occur when changing from one system speed to another?

_____

_____

4. **Based on your results, what general rule can you synthesize regarding screen speed and detail/sharpness?**

_____

_____

_____

5. **Evaluate the computed radiography image compared to the film-based image that you selected as the most optimal:**

Is the sharpness of the CR image higher or lower? _____

How does a CR-based system differ from a film-based system that would explain this difference in detail?

_____

_____

_____

Processing: Time Versus Temperature

Name: _____ Date: _____

Optimum processing conditions are important to ensure the final diagnostic quality of radiographic films. Even if positioning and technique selection are perfect, improper processing can ruin the image and cause a repeat exposure.

Three factors that control the quality of the chemicals used in the processor are time, temperature, and concentration. Varying any or all of these will have observable effects on the radiographic image because of their effects on density, contrast, and fog.

Objectives:

Upon completion of this lab, the student will be able to:

1. Demonstrate the proper method to measure developer temperature.
2. Demonstrate the proper operation of a sensitometer and densitometer.
3. Demonstrate and describe the effect of increased developing time on radiographic density, contrast, and fog.
4. Demonstrate and describe the effect of increased developing temperature on radiographic density, contrast, and fog.

Materials:

1. Film processor
2. Sensitometer
3. Thermometer (not glass)
4. 8 × 10-in radiographic film
5. Densitometer

Procedure:

1. In the darkroom with the white light off, write the number "1" on a sheet of 8 × 10-in film using a lead pencil. Expose the film in the sensitometer.

2. Record the developer temperature using the thermometer.

3. Turn on a processor that has not been running for some time (the temperature should be less than optimal for this segment of the lab). Immediately process film no. 1.

4. Wait for the developer temperature in the processor to reach normal levels. Repeat Step no. 1, but mark the film as no. 2.

5. Repeat Step no. 1, but mark the next film as no. 3.

6. Feed film no. 3 into the processor. Exactly 10 seconds after the trailing end of the film has entered the processor, turn the processor off for 90 seconds. At the end of 90 seconds, turn the processor back on.

7. Using a densitometer, measure the ODs of the steps for film no. 2. Find the step closest to 1 + B + F; this will be used as the film's speed step. Record this step's density and the film's B + F density; record these steps' densities for films nos. 1 and 3 also. (See the table below.)

8. Measure the OD of the step two steps darker than the speed step for film no. 2. This value will be used to help determine the film's contrast. Repeat for films nos. 1 and 3.

9. Shut the processor off as soon as your films are completed for the next group, if applicable.

Data:

	Reference Step		
	Film No. 1	Film No. 2	Film No. 3
Developer temperature	_____	_____	_____
B + F (Step no. _____)	_____	_____	_____
OD of speed step (Step no._____)	_____	_____	_____
OD of step that is two steps darker (Step no._____)	_____	_____	_____
Contrast value (difference between the two steps)	_____	_____	_____

Analysis:

1. **Visually evaluate the three images. Identify the image that displays the:**

    a. Highest B + F: _____   Lowest B + F: _____
    b. Highest density: _____   Lowest density: _____
    c. Highest contrast: _____   Lowest contrast: _____

2. **Using your measurements above, identify the image that displays the:**

    a. Highest B + F: _____   Lowest B + F: _____
    b. Highest density: _____   Lowest density: _____
    c. Highest contrast: _____   Lowest contrast: _____

3. Did your visual inspection agree with the calculated findings? If not, explain.

_____

_____

_____

4. Based on your results, what effect does processing time have on radiographic quality and temperature? (Be sure to address all of the image qualities that apply.)

Time:

_____

_____

Temperature:

_____

_____

5. How could these findings be put to practical use for processor quality control purposes?

_____

_____

_____

6. Modern automatic film processors complete the development stage of the film processing sequence in approximately 20 seconds, while manual processing requires 3 to 5 minutes for complete development. Explain why these times are so different.

_____

_____

_____

Effect of Source-to-Image Receptor Distance on Magnification and Image Detail

Name: _____   Date: _____

Changes in the source-to-image receptor distance (SID) affect image density, along with geometric properties of the image: specifically detail and magnification. Generally, the longest SID possible should be used because less penumbra results and magnification is minimized or eliminated. This lab provides students with the opportunity to observe and measure the effects of SID on magnification and detail.

Objectives:

Upon completion of this lab, the student will be able to:

1. Use and interpret a line pair resolution test tool pattern.
2. Evaluate radiographic images with different SIDs.
3. Analyze the effects of a changed SID on magnification.
4. Analyze the effects of a changed SID on image detail.

Materials:

1. A small dry bone, such as a phalanx
2. Line pair resolution test pattern (lp/mm)
3. 3 to 4-in sponge
4. Ruler or tape measure
5. 14 × 17-in image receptor
6. Lead numbers

Procedure:

1. Place the small dry bone and the line resolution test pattern on the sponge on top of the image receptor using a 36 in SID (Exposure no. 1). Expose using 54 kVp at 0.15 mAs (or another technique that demonstrates adequate density).

2. For Exposure no. 2, place the dry bone and line resolution test pattern on the sponge on top of the image receptor using a 72 in SID (Exposure no. 2). Expose using 54 kVp at 0.6 mAs (or another technique that demonstrates adequate density).

3. Using a ruler, measure the length of the bone (in cm) and record where indicated.

4. Analyze the line pair resolution test pattern measurements for each exposure. Record the lp/mm measurement in the Data Table.

5. Using a ruler, measure the length of the bone (in cm) for each exposure. Record each measurement in the Data Table.

6. Calculate the magnification factor of each image by using the formula: MF = image bone length/actual bone length. Record in the appropriate column of the Data Table.

7. Analyze the images and answer the questions as indicated.

Data:

Original bone length: _____ (cm)

Exposure No.	SID (in)	Resolution (lp/mm)	Image Bone Length (cm)	Magnification Factor
1				
2				

Analysis:

1. Visually analyze the edges and the bony trabeculae of each image. Which exposure appears to have the sharpest detail?

_____

_____

_____

2. Compare the lp/mm readings of each exposure. According to your data, which exposure has the highest detail (i.e., highest lp/mm)?

a. Does this agree with your visual analysis? Why or why not?

_____

_____

_____

3. Compare the bone length measurements and the magnification factor calculations for each exposure. According to your data, which exposure caused the most magnification?

_____

_____

_____

4. Based on your results, complete the following sentence by selecting and inserting the appropriate answer: "To produce radiographs with the highest detail and minimum magnification, a(n) _____ (decreased/increased) SID should be used."

Effect of Object-to-Image Receptor Distance on Magnification and Image Detail

Name: _____   Date: _____

The object-to-image receptor distance (OID) plays a major role in size distortion, or magnification, and affects the amount of image blur present in an image. Generally, the shortest OID possible should be used so that less penumbra is produced and magnification is minimized or eliminated. This lab provides students with the opportunity to observe and measure the effects of OID on magnification and detail.

Objectives:

Upon completion of this lab, the student will be able to:

1. Use and interpret a line pair resolution test tool pattern.
2. Evaluate radiographic images with different OIDs.
3. Analyze the effects of a changed OID on magnification.
4. Analyze the effects of a changed OID on image detail.

Materials:

1. A small dry bone, such as a phalanx
2. Line pair resolution test pattern (lp/mm)
3. One 1-in sponge and two 3 to 4-in sponges
4. Ruler or tape measure
5. 14 × 17-in image receptor
6. Lead numbers

Procedure:

1. Place the small dry bone directly on the image receptor and the line resolution test pattern on the 1-in sponge directly beside it. Place on top of the image receptor using a 40 in SID. (Exposure no. 1) Expose using 56 kVp at 0.15 mAs (or another technique that demonstrates adequate density). Maintain this technique for all three exposures.

2. For Exposure no. 2, place both the dry bone and line resolution test pattern on the 3-4-inch sponge on top of the image receptor. Maintain a 40 in SID.

3. For Exposure no. 3, place the two 3 to 4-in sponges on top of each other to create an OID of 6 to 8 in. Place both the dry bone and line resolution test pattern on top of both sponges. Maintain the 40 in SID.

4. Using a ruler, measure the length of the bone (in cm) and record where indicated.

5. Analyze the line pair resolution test pattern measurements for each exposure. Record the lp/mm measurement in the Data Table.

6. Using a ruler, measure the length of the bone (in cm) for each exposure. Record each measurement in the Data Table.

7. Calculate the magnification factor of each image by using the formula: MF = image bone length/actual bone length. Record in the appropriate column of the Data Table.

8. Analyze the images and answer the questions as indicated.

Data:

Original bone length: _____ (cm)

Exposure No.	OID (in)	Resolution (lp/mm)	Image Bone Length (cm)	Magnification Factor
1				
2				
3				

Analysis:

1. Visually analyze the edges and the bony trabeculae of each image. Which exposure appears to have the sharpest detail and which one has the least detail?

_____

_____

_____

2. Compare the lp/mm readings of each exposure. According to your data, which exposure has the highest detail (i.e., highest lp/mm) and which one the least detail?

   a. Does this agree with your visual analysis? Why or why not?

   _____

   _____

   _____

3. Compare the bone length measurements and the magnification factor calculations for each exposure. According to your data, which exposure caused the most magnification?

   _____

   _____

   _____

4. Based on your results, complete the following sentence by selecting and inserting the appropriate answer: "To produce radiographs with the highest detail and minimum magnification, a(n) _____ (decreased/increased) OID should be used."

Effect of Grids on Radiographic Density and Contrast

Name: _____ **Date:** _____

A grid is a radiographic device made of alternating strips of lead and radiolucent materials used to absorb scatter radiation before it reaches the image receptor. The lead strips work to absorb the scatter radiation, while the radiolucent strips allow the more forward traveling photons through to the image receptor. When scatter radiation is absorbed, density is lost (if no technique compensation is made), but there is a significant improvement in image contrast. There are various grid ratios available. In order to maintain density when changing from nongrid to a grid exposure, or from grid to grid, the following formula is used:

$$mAs_2 = mAs_1 \, (GCF_2)/(GCF_1)$$

This lab provides students with the opportunity to observe and measure the effects of nongrid and grid exposures on radiographic density and contrast.

Objectives:

Upon completion of this lab, the student will be able to:

1. Convert techniques to compensate for changes in grid ratio.
2. Visually evaluate radiographs for changes in density and contrast when different grids are used.
3. Evaluate changes in density and contrast using the densitometer and calculations when grid changes are made.

Materials:

1. Energized x-ray unit
2. Abdomen or pelvis phantom
3. Three grids of varying grid ratios (10 × 12 in or 14 × 17 in)
4. Densitometer
5. Lead markers

Procedure:

1. Place the pelvis phantom in an AP position directly on a 10 × 12-in cassette (or 14 × 17 in, consistent with the grid sizes) for the no grid exposure. Place the central ray at the level of the ASIS and centered to the spine. Number the exposure as Exposure no. 1 and expose the image using the following recommended technique: 80 kVp at 5 mAs or a suitable technique to provide adequate density.

2. Convert your Exposure no. 1 technique using the grid conversion factor formula for the three grid ratios chosen. (NOTE: The suggested Bucky or grid conversion factors to use for each grid can be found in Table 12.1 of the text book).

3. For Exposure no. 2, place the grid tube side up on top of the cassette. Place the phantom on top of the grid, centering exactly the same as Exposure no. 1.

4. Repeat Step 3 for the remaining two grid ratios.

5. After the films are exposed and processed, circle two homogenous densities: one a darker density in an area of soft tissue (Area A) and one a lighter density in an area of bony anatomy (Area B).

6. Measure the densities of Area A and Area B for each film and complete the Data Table where indicated.

7. To calculate contrast for each image, divide the density of Area A by the density of Area B (A/B). Complete the appropriate column on the Data Table.

8. Analyze the images and answer the questions as indicated.

Data:

Exposure No.	Grid Ratio	mAs	Area A Density	Area B Density	Contrast (A/B)
1					
2					
3					
4					

Analysis:

1. **Visually compare the densities of all four exposures. Was density maintained for all four exposures?**

   a. If not, for which exposures were density not maintained?

   _____

   _____

   _____

2. **Compare the density readings for Area A for all four exposures. Find the average of all four density readings by adding them together and dividing by four:**

   a. Average density for Area A: _____

   _____

   _____

   _____

   b. To find an acceptable density range, multiply the average density for Area A by 0.25 (25%). Add and subtract this value from the average density value:

   i. Acceptable range of densities: _____ to _____

   Average density – 25%   Average density + 25%

   _____

   _____

   _____

   c. Do all of the density values fall within the acceptable range of densities?

   _____

   _____

   _____

d. In other words, did the technique changes compensate for the grid change? If not, what technique(s) (or mAs) do you feel would have worked better? (HINT: Use your density readings to help you determine this.)

_____

_____

_____

3. Visually evaluate all of the images. Which image appears to have the highest contrast and which one has the lowest?

_____

_____

_____

4. Evaluate your contrast values in the Data Table. Based on your calculations, which image exhibits the highest contrast and which one the lowest? Does this agree with your visual analysis? Why or why not?

_____

_____

_____

5. Note your contrast values again. What is the purpose of adding a grid?

_____

_____

_____

6. What generalization can be made regarding the relationship between increasing grid ratios and contrast?

_____

_____

_____

Fluoroscopy and C-arms: Components of Image Intensified Fluoroscopy Systems

Name: _____   Date: _____

Fluoroscopy is a dynamic imaging modality designed to observe moving structures in the body, in contrast to conventional radiography that produces static images of body structures. This imaging method allows the radiologist or other physicians to observe physiological functions and the proper placement of medical devices during surgical procedures. The technologist is often called to assist and/or operate the fluoroscope, so it is important that he or she be knowledgeable of the controls and functions of this device.

Objectives:

Upon completion of this lab, the student will be able to:

1. Identify the controls of a stationary fluoroscope and describe their functions.
2. Identify the controls of a mobile fluoroscope and describe their functions.
3. Compare and contrast the controls and functions of a stationary and mobile fluoroscope.
4. Describe the imaging chain, listing all of the energy conversions that occur prior to obtaining a visible image.

Materials:

1. A stationary fluoroscopic unit (and operator's manual, if needed)
2. A mobile fluoroscopic unit (and operator's manual, if needed)

Procedure:

1. Follow the instructions and answer the questions provided.

Part A

Data and Analysis:

Below is a diagram of a patient on a radiographic examination table. Draw and label the following components:

1. X-ray tube
2. Image intensifier
3. Carriage or "C-arm"
4. Video camera tube or CCD
5. Monitor

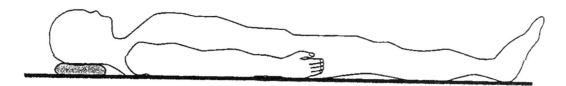

Answer the following questions based on your drawing and the information covered in the textbook:

1. Where is the source of radiation located in reference to the patient?

_____

_____

_____

2. If a gonad shield was used, where should it be placed to protect the patient?

_____

_____

_____

3. Where is the "image receptor" in this case?

_____

_____

_____

4. Trace the imaging chain from the x-ray tube (primary radiation) to the monitor (visible light) by listing the components traveled through and the conversions made from one form of energy to another.

_____

_____

_____

Part B:

Data and Analysis:

1. Diagram and label the operator's panel of a stationary fluoroscopy unit below.

2. Underneath your diagram, briefly describe the function of each button or switch.

_____

_____

_____

Part C:
Data and Analysis:

1. Diagram and label the operator's panel of a mobile fluoroscopy unit (C-arm) below.

2. Underneath your diagram, briefly describe the function of each button or switch.

_____

_____

_____

3. List the similarities of the two units' controls and functions, along with any differences where indicated below:

Similarities	Differences
_____	_____
_____	_____
_____	_____

Fluoroscopy and C-arm Use: Fluoroscopic Image Quality and the Automatic Brightness Control System

Name: _____   Date: _____

Fluoroscopy is a dynamic imaging modality that allows live moving structures to be imaged and observed. Although this imaging method allows the direct observation of physiological functions, radiographic image quality is sacrificed. Because the fluoroscope is often moved during a procedure, the unit must be able to compensate for changes in body thickness, so that each body structure can be visualized during the examination. The device that allows this to occur is called the Automatic Brightness Control System.

This lab will provide students with the opportunity to operate a stationary and/or mobile fluoroscopic system, evaluate the quality of the images produced, and observe the operation of the Automatic Brightness Control System during fluoroscopy.

Objectives:

Upon completion of this lab, the student will be able to:

1. Safely operate a stationary or mobile fluoroscope.
2. Determine the technical factors typically used during fluoroscopy.
3. Evaluate the radiographic quality of fluoroscopic images.
4. Describe the effects of Automatic Brightness Control on the image during fluoroscopy.

Materials:

1. A stationary or mobile fluoroscopic unit (and operator's manual, if needed)
2. A radiographic examination table
3. Hip, shoulder, thorax, or abdominal phantom
4. Lead aprons

Procedure:

1. Have everyone who will be participating in the lab put on a lead apron.

2. Perform the necessary start-up procedures for the fluoroscopy unit.

3. Under supervision, operate the fluoroscope as described and answer the questions provided.

Data and Analysis:

Place the phantom underneath the image intensifier of a stationary or mobile fluoroscopy unit. Have one person operate the fluoro, and another at the control panel to note the conditions of the exposure. Depress the exposure switch briefly, while noting the following:

1. **List the technical factors (kVp/mA/time) and their settings that are displayed while the fluoro is engaged.**

   a. How do the technical factors you listed above compare to conventional overhead techniques?

   _____

   _____

   _____

2. **While fluoroscopy is in progress, what indicator(s) is (are) present that the fluoro is "on"?**

   _____

   _____

   _____

   Begin fluoro again. While watching the monitor, open and close the collimators.

3. **Describe what changes occurred in the image in terms of density (brightness), contrast, and noise/fog when the collimators were changed.**

   _____

   _____

   _____

4. Overall, in terms of sharpness of detail, how does the image on the monitor compare with the same image if it were a static radiographic image?

_____

_____

_____

5. View the image on the monitor again, both from a normal viewing distance and up close to the screen. You should note that the image appears grainy. What is the radiographic term for this quality? What causes it to occur?

_____

_____

_____

Resume fluoro again, moving the carriage so that the phantom is centered to the image. Move the carriage and/or table slowly from the center of the phantom to one side, observing the image closely during the motion. Return the carriage slowly to the center of the phantom, and then move it (or the table) gradually up or down until the phantom disappears from the image.

6. Describe how the image changes as the fluoroscope moves from a thick portion of the phantom to a thin region.

_____

_____

_____

7. Identify the mechanism that causes the changes in Question no. 6, and briefly describe how it works.

_____

_____

_____

Digital Imaging: Effects on Radiographic Quality

Name: _____ Date: _____

The processes used by digital imaging systems to acquire and view a radiographic image are significantly different than conventional film/screen systems. As a result, significant changes are also noted in the radiographic qualities of density (brightness), contrast, noise, and detail. In addition, digital imaging processes also affect how technical factor changes are demonstrated on the image as compared to conventional film/screen images. This lab provides students with the opportunity to compare the radiographic qualities of a film/screen image with a digital image and to evaluate changes in a digital radiographic image and exposure indicator numbers when various technical factors are changed.

Objectives:

Upon completion of this lab, the student will be able to:

1. Correctly expose and interpret a resolution test pattern tool.
2. Evaluate density, contrast, noise, detail, magnification, and distortion of a radiographic film image and a digital image.
3. Compare the radiographic qualities of a radiographic film image and a digital image.
4. Evaluate the exposure indicator number of a digital image.
5. Describe the effects of various technique changes on a digital radiographic image.
6. Use a digital imaging system's postprocessing tools to manipulate a digital radiographic image.
7. Determine which technique errors are able to be corrected using postprocessing tools and/ or which errors require a repeat exposure.

Materials:

1. Energized x-ray unit
2. Hand phantom
3. One 8 × 10 -in or 10 × 12 -in film cassette
4. Automatic processor
5. Digital imaging unit (CR or DR)
6. Line pair resolution tool
7. 1-in positioning sponge
8. Lead markers to number exposures

Part I:

Procedure:

1. Expose a phantom hand using a radiographic film/screen extremity cassette, setting a technique to obtain a diagnostic quality radiograph. Place a resolution test pattern on a 1-in sponge next to the hand. Make the exposure and process the film under normal processing conditions. Technique: _____

2. Repeat the exposure with a CR imaging plate or DR system using the normal hand technique for that unit. Process the image. Note the Exposure Indicator Number where indicated in the Data Table. Technique: _____

3. Expose the phantom and resolution test pattern again using the CR imaging plate, but use two times the mAs. Record your results.

4. Exposure no. 4: Return to the original technique. Using the 15% rule, decrease the kVp and expose the phantom and test pattern again.

5. Repeat Exposure no. 2. When processing the image, select something other than the hand algorithm (i.e., select another body part).

Data:

Exposure No.	Technique (kVp/mAs)	Exposure Indicator Number	Resolution (lp/mm)

1. **Compare Exposures 1 and 2 and your data in the Data Table. Which exposure provides the highest: (Answer "N" if neither appears to be higher in the listed radiographic quality.)**

_____ Density?   _____ Detail?

_____ Contrast?   _____ Magnification?

_____ Noise?   _____ Distortion?

a. Which exposure, Exposure no. 1 or 2, resolved the highest detail? Explain possible reasons for this:

_____

_____

_____

2. Compare and describe the indicated radiographic quality(ies) of the images obtained in Exposures 3 and 4 with Exposures 1 and 2:

   a. Density:

   _____

   _____

   _____

   b. Contrast:

   _____

   _____

   _____

   c. Detail:

   _____

   _____

   _____

   d. Which, if any, of the exposures were able to be corrected? Explain why the image was able/not able to be corrected in each situation.

   _____

   _____

   _____

3. Compare the Exposure Indicator Numbers of Exposures 2, 3, and 4. What does the Exposure Number seem to indicate about the following?

   a. The exposure received by the imaging plate/receptor

   _____

   _____

   _____

b. The detail resolved in each case

_____

_____

_____

c. The overall quality of the radiographic image

_____

_____

_____

4. **Identify the algorithm chosen for Exposure no. 5:** _____

Describe the radiographic quality(ies) of the image obtained in Exposure no. 5:

Density:

_____

_____

Contrast:

_____

_____

Noise:

_____

_____

Detail:

_____

_____

a. How did the Exposure Indicator Number compare to Exposure no. 2?

_____

_____

_____

b. Is this error able to be corrected by changing the window level or width? If not, what must the technologist do?

_____

_____

_____

5. Based on your observations, which of the following imaging and positioning factors in digital radiography are still the responsibility of the technologist? (Check all that apply.)

_____ kVp selection   _____ mAs selection

_____ Photocell selection   _____ Grid use

_____ Anatomic part selection   _____ SID selection

_____ Appropriate centering   _____ Correct positioning

_____ R and L markers   _____ Patient identification

_____ Collimation   _____ Patient instructions

Part II: Analyzing the Digital Imaging Chain

1. Identify two similarities between a film/screen cassette and how it is processed, and the CR imaging plate and how it is "processed." What are two differences between the two?

_____

_____

_____

2. Why is it usually not a good idea to place more than one exposure on an imaging plate (i.e., all three wrist views on one plate), even though this has been a recognized routine in most departments using film/screens? Explain how performing the "original" routine affects the digital processing of the images in your answer.

_____

_____

_____

3. Once an image has been "processed" by the laser reader or electronically, what happens to the image next? (Where does it go, etc.?)

_____

_____

_____

4. List three advantages of digital imaging over traditional film/screen systems.

_____

_____

_____

5. Is a system like this totally error-free? If not, what do you think are two to three primary errors that the technologist is most likely to make using this system?

_____

_____

_____

Digital Radiography Quality Control: Image Integrity

Name: _____   Date: _____

The advantages that digital imaging systems have over conventional film/screen systems include a wide dynamic range, increased contrast resolution, and the ability to postprocess an image after exposure. However, the workstations and monitors used by the technologist are significantly different than the workstations and monitors used by the radiologist for diagnosis. Due to this, any windowing completed by technologists at their workstations can have a significant effect on the image and its diagnostic value if these changes are saved prior to sending them to the radiologist or diagnosing physician for interpretation.

This lab provides the opportunity for students to observe and compare the images at different workstations and the effects that postprocessing can have on the diagnostic value of the image.

Objectives:

Upon completion of this lab, the student will be able to:

1. Compare the differences in resolution between the workstations and monitors in the general work area with those used by the radiologist for diagnosis.
2. Complete basic postprocessing and windowing of a digital image.
3. Observe the effects of windowing an image on workstations and monitors in the general work area on the image sent to the high-resolution monitor used by the radiologist.
4. Describe and compare some of the postprocessing tools and functions available on workstations in the general work area and on the radiologist's high-resolution monitor.
5. Explain the importance of maintaining the integrity of and sending the original exposed image to the radiologist or interpreting physician without saving postprocessing changes.

Materials:

1. Two digital images, preferably on phantoms or images that are not being used for diagnostic purposes
2. General diagnostic monitor and workstation
3. High-resolution monitor and workstation

Procedure:

1. Consult with a technologist prior to conducting this lab, ensuring the availability of the radiologist's high-resolution monitor and the creation of an artificial patient file for the images being used/created for this laboratory.

2. Follow the instructions and answer the questions.

Data and Analysis:

Before sending a completed radiographic procedure to PACS for diagnosis to the radiologist or interpreting physician, each image must be checked for diagnostic quality.

1. Provide a list of the items checked on each image prior to it being sent electronically for interpretation. Beside each item, describe its parameters and/or guidelines for acceptance.

_____

_____

_____

Generally, the imaging workstations used by the radiologists have a larger matrix, greater contrast resolution capability, and a greater capacity to enhance and manipulate images than the workstations used by the technologists.

2. Observe and enhance a digital radiography image at both workstations.

   NOTE: Do NOT save your image enhancements prior to sending it to the radiologist's workstation.

   a. Which workstation appears to have a greater contrast resolution?

   _____

   _____

   _____

   b. Which workstation appears to have a higher detail?

   _____

   _____

   _____

c. What image enhancement tools are available on the radiologists' workstation that are NOT available on the technologists'?

_____

_____

_____

d. Utilize some of the image enhancement tools listed. How do the image enhancement tools listed above change the image?

_____

_____

_____

e. Which workstation images do you feel are more diagnostic? Why?

_____

_____

_____

3. Observe and enhance a digital radiography image at both workstations.

NOTE: This time, SAVE your image enhancements prior to sending it to the radiologist's workstation.

a. View the image on the radiologists' workstation. Does it appear different than the first image you sent? Explain.

_____

_____

_____

b. Utilize some of the same image enhancement tools you used above. Describe any changes you notice in the image and/or your ability to manipulate the image compared to your first image.

_____

_____

_____

4. Based on your observations and results, if a digital image has an acceptable exposure indicator number, what image enhancements should a technologist perform on an image prior to sending it for interpretation?

_____

_____

_____

Digital Imaging Artifacts

Name: _____   **Date:** _____

The conversion from conventional film/screen radiography to digital imaging has not been without its problems. Traditional routines (such as more than one projection per cassette) may not provide the optimal diagnostic images needed, and even though there is no longer a physical film, the image receptor and the other equipment used to obtain a radiographic image may still create artifacts or other unwanted information.

Objectives:

Upon completion of this lab, the student will be able to:

1. List some of the causes of radiographic artifacts when digital imaging is used.
2. Identify and describe the artifact(s) specific to the imaging problem created during CR/DR use.
3. Describe the corrective action(s) necessary to eliminate the artifact(s) identified.
4. Implement the corrective action(s) identified, as applicable.

Procedure:

1. Select one CR or DR problem/incorrect protocol specific to digital imaging from the list below.

2. Using an appropriate phantom and technique, expose the phantom using the correct CR/DR protocol.

3. For your next exposure(s), expose the same phantom using the incorrect protocol you selected.

4. Answer the questions provided.

Digital Imaging Problems/Incorrect Protocols

- Placing more than one exposure on one imaging plate

- Placing more than one anatomical part on the detector

- No collimated borders visible on the imaging plate

- Using a grid with a frequency in the range of 100 lines/in

- Leaving an imaging plate in the room while other exposures are made

- Exposing an imaging plate upside down

- Collimating down so that <20% of the imaging plate is exposed

- Exposing anatomy with a metal artifact in place (e.g., a surgically implanted pin or nail)

- Displaying four visible collimation borders, but noticeably off-centered on the plate (the anatomy off-centered OR the entire field itself)

Protocol Error Selected: _____

Anatomy/Phantom Used: _____   X-ray Unit Used: _____

Technique Used: _____   Exposure Indicator No.: _____

Exercises:

1. **Evaluate the radiographic image exposed under optimum conditions using the appropriate terms:**

   Image Brightness: _____   Contrast: _____

   Noise: _____   Exposure Indicator No.: _____

   Other Indicators:

   _____

   _____

2. **Evaluate the radiographic image exposed using the incorrect image protocol chosen:**

   Image Brightness: _____   Contrast: _____

   Noise: _____   Exposure Indicator No.: _____

   Other Indicators:

   _____

   _____

Describe the artifact(s)/image problem created:

_____

_____

3. Which indicator(s) in Question no. 2 above served as the primary cue that the digital image was not adequate? Explain how this indicator was affected.

_____

_____

_____

4. If the incorrectly exposed image had been taken on an actual patient, explain how it would have to be corrected.

_____

_____

_____

5. Which computed radiography image/equipment/software function(s) and/or components were "misled" by the erroneous exposure conditions?

_____

_____

_____

6. How can the artifact(s)/image problem you created be prevented from occurring?

_____

_____

_____

Field Size and Beam Alignment Quality Control

Name: _____   Date: _____

Radiographic quality control consists of periodic monitoring of the x-ray tube, the accuracy of the exposure factors, and the collimation device. Regular quality control tests can detect problems with equipment before they cause repeat exposures; they can also be performed to help determine the cause of an imaging problem.

It is important that the light field and radiation field coincide so that the x-ray field placement is correct. This ensures that only the desired anatomy is irradiated and that the entire desired anatomy is imaged. Federal guidelines require that the light field size and x-ray field size match with a variance of only ±2% of the SID allowed. Each side of the x-ray field and light field, in addition to the central ray placement, must be congruent to within ±1% of the SID.

Objectives:

Upon completion of this lab, the student will be able to:

1. Use the appropriate measurement tools for a field size quality control test.
2. Evaluate and measure the light field size and the actual x-ray field size.
3. Analyze the results and determine the compliance of the x-ray unit tested with federal requirements regarding collimation and field size.

Materials:

1. Energized x-ray unit.
2. Film cassette and automatic processor (or the ability to print a digital image to scale)
3. Field size and CR alignment device (or paper clips/pennies)

Procedure:

1. Place the field size alignment device on the cassette, collimating to the indicated borders (or collimate to a smaller field than the cassette size and mark off the borders of the light field using paper clips or pennies).

2. Note the collimator setting and measure the actual size of the light field and record below.

3. Mark each edge of the light field as North, South, East, and West.

4. Expose the cassette using approximately an ankle technique. SID: 40 in (100 cm)

5. Process or print the image.

6. Record each measurement as instructed and answer the questions provided.

Data and Analysis:

1. **Note the collimator setting and measure the actual size of the light field on the cassette.**

   a. Collimator setting: Length = _____(in or cm)
                              Width = _____ (in or cm)
   b. Light field: Length = _____(in or cm)
                              Width = _____ (in or cm)

2. **Measure the actual x-ray field and record below:**

   a. X-ray field: Length = _____(in or cm)
                              Width = _____ (in or cm)

3. **How much variance is allowed between the indicated light field size and the x-ray field size?**

   _____

   _____

   _____

4. **Does this unit meet this standard? Explain.**

   _____

   _____

   _____

5. **For each edge of the x-ray field, measure how far the edge of the x-ray field (black exposed area) is from the light field markers and in which direction. List your results below:**

   a. North side = _____ cm off to _____ (direction)
   b. South side = _____ cm off to _____ (direction)
   c. East side   = _____ cm off to _____ (direction)
   d. West side = _____ cm off to _____ (direction)

6. Divide each of the deviation measurements in number 5 above by the SID (100 cm) and multiply this result by 100 to obtain the percentage deviation from the SID and record below:

   a. North side = _____ % of SID off
   b. South side = _____ % of SID off
   c. East side = _____ % of SID off
   d. West side = _____ % of SID off

7. How much variance is allowed for each side of the light field alignment from the actual x-ray field?

   _____

   _____

   _____

8. Which, if any, of the light field edges are out of alignment by unacceptable amounts?

   _____

   _____

   _____

9. To determine the accuracy of the central ray alignment, draw diagonal lines from each pair of corners of both the black x-ray field and the light field (as outlined by the field size device or the paper clips or pennies). Each "X" formed represents the location of its respective "central ray." Measure with a ruler the distance from the x-ray field central ray to the light field central ray and note in which direction it is off and record below:

   a. Light field center is _____ cm off toward _____ (direction) from x-ray field center.

   _____

   _____

   _____

10. Divide this measurement by the SID (100 cm) and multiply the result times 100 to obtain the percentage of deviation from the SID and record below:

    a. Light field center is _____ % of SID off of alignment.

    _____

    _____

    _____

11. How much variance is allowed for the central ray placement from the light field center?

_____

_____

_____

12. Is your answer in Question number 10 in compliance with this standard?

_____

_____

_____

Digital Radiography Quality Control Activity Log

Name: _____ **Date:** _____

A digital imaging department's components require regular quality control monitoring to ensure diagnostic quality images. These include (1) the laser reader, (2) the image display workstation, (3) the computed radiography (CR) and digital radiography (DR) imaging equipment/imaging plates, and (4) the picture archiving communication system. This lab provides the student with the opportunity to observe and participate in the quality control of the department.

Objectives:

Upon completion of this lab, the student will be able to:

1. List the various QC actions taken on a daily, monthly, or other systematic basis in a digital imaging environment.
2. Explain the importance of conducting regular QC testing of digital imaging equipment.
3. Describe the QC actions taken regarding the care and maintenance of imaging plates, a DR system, the PACS network, and the image display workstation.
4. Observe and participate in available CR/DR QC activities.

Procedure:

During a period of 1 month or other monitoring period as designated by your instructor, you will be

1. Investigating what regular QC tests are conducted in a digital imaging department and/or discovering what additional tests may be completed, document your results by completing the table and answering the questions in Part I of this lab.

2. Documenting the results of your participation in various QC activities, complete the table in Part II of this lab and answer the questions.

Part I: Digital Imaging QC Activities
Data and Analysis:

1. What activities are conducted by the department to ensure the accurate acquisition and display of images on the imaging plates and the imaging workstations? Complete the table below as indicated.

   NOTE: You may have already observed some of these activities; others you may need to obtain by interviewing the department's designated PACS/QC personnel.

CR Component: QC Action or Test	Accuracy Requirements	Frequency	Who Conducts/ Other Information
CR PLATES 1.			
2.			
VIDEO MONITOR/ WORKSTATION			
1.			
2.			
LASER READER, PRINTER, AND/ OR PACS SYSTEM			
1.			
2.			

2. After completing the table, select ONE item from EACH category and explain how the completion of this test or activity ensures an optimum image and/or maintains the optimal operation of the system/department. (i.e., What would happen if this activity was NOT completed?)

_____

_____

_____

_____

_____

Part II: QC Activity Log
Data and Analysis:

1. During the QC period, you will need to document your participation in and/or observation of various CR/DR/PACS QC activities. It is desirable that you participate in as many of these activities as possible. However, a one-time demonstration of some of the activities conducted on a less frequent basis is also acceptable. Log your activities on the attached table to be turned in at the end of the period.

Log of Quality Control Activities

During the QC period, document your observation of and/or **participation** in the department's QC activities using the table below.

Date	Activity	Observed or Participated	Date	Activity	Observed or Participated

Summary

1. Which activities did you engage in the most?

_____

_____

_____

2. List any problems you encountered and/or potential problems you were able to prevent due to your activities.

_____

_____

_____

3. Briefly describe your impressions of the state of QC in radiology with regard to DR, CR, and PACS as a result of this lab activity.

_____

_____

_____

Repeat/Reject Analysis

Name: _____ Date: _____

An important component of a quality control program is monitoring repeat exposures and reject images. By identifying trends in repeat/reject exposures, a department can determine the causes of the repeat or reject exposures and take steps to correct the identified problems. By eliminating repeat exposures, a department can save time and money, and reduce patient exposure. This lab provides students with the opportunity to track and analyze their own repeat or reject exposures.

Objectives:

Upon completion of this lab, the student will be able to:

1. Calculate his or her repeat rate for the entire period.
2. Calculate his or her repeat rate by cause.
3. Calculate his or her repeat rate by exam category.
4. Identify trends and possible causes of his or her repeat exposures.
5. Synthesize strategies and solutions to improve his or her repeat rate.

Materials:

1. Daily Procedure Record (additional copies may need to be made to cover the full reporting period)
2. Repeat Analysis Worksheet
3. Calculator

Procedure:

1. For a period of 1 month, or as directed by your instructor, record all of your repeat radiographs regardless of cause.

2. During this time period, keep accurate records of the total number of views taken, completing Chart A (Daily Procedure Record) for every procedure. (Note: You are to record the number of exposures or views taken, not simply the number of films/imaging plates used.)

3. At the end of the data collection period, complete Chart B (Repeat Analysis Worksheet) by transferring the total number of exposures (views) taken each day into appropriate categories. Add the totals together as directed to determine the grand total for the period in each period.

4. Answer the questions as indicated.

Results and Analysis:

1. Total your Daily Procedure Record. Record the grand total number of views taken here:_____

2. Record the total number of repeat exposures made here: _____

3. To calculate your overall repeat rate, divide the total number of repeat exposures taken for the period by the grand total number of views. Multiply the result by 100.

   Overall repeat rate: _____%

4. Next, examine and tally the primary causes of your repeats and sort into each of the categories below. Record the number of repeats in each group:

Reason for Repeat	Number of Repeats
Positioning	_____
Overexposed	_____
Underexposed	_____
Motion	_____
Artifacts on the patient, film, or table/processing	_____
Other: Collimation or alignment (centering)	_____
TOTAL:	_____

5. Compute your causal repeat rate as follows: Divide the number of repeats for each reason by the total number of repeats for the period. Multiply the result by 100. Record your repeat rate for each category below:

Positioning	_____%
Overexposed	_____%
Underexposed	_____%
Motion	_____%
Artifacts on the patient, film, or table/processing	_____%
Other: Collimation or alignment (centering)	_____%

6. Which type of problem caused the most repeat exposures and which type the second-most?

_____

_____

_____

7. If you were a supervisor, what actions would you initiate in your department to reduce the type of repeats listed above if this was a department-wide problem? (Think of at least two different strategies to ensure improvement.)

_____

_____

_____

8. Next, look over your Repeat Analysis Worksheet to evaluate your repeats by exam category. To calculate your repeat rate, divide the number of repeats taken for each procedure by the total number of repeats for the period. Multiply each result by 100% and record in the % column on the far right of the Worksheet.

_____

_____

_____

9. Which exams/procedures had the highest repeat rate and which ones the second highest?

_____

_____

_____

10. If you were a supervisor, what actions would you initiate in your department to reduce the type of repeats listed above if this was a department-wide problem? (Think of at least two different strategies to ensure improvement.)

_____

_____

_____

Chart A: Daily Procedure Record

For each date of data collection, complete each column calculating the number of views expected and actually taken.

Date	Exam	Routine No. of Views Taken	Actual No. of Views Taken	No. or Views Repeated/Cause
	Total for this date:			

Date	Exam	Routine No. of Views Taken	Actual No. of Views Taken	No. or Views Repeated/Cause
	Total for this date:			

Chart B: Repeat Analysis Worksheet

Using the Daily Procedure Record, complete the chart below filling in the total number of exposures (views) taken in each exam category. Assign procedures taken into the categories shown as follows:

Torso	Head	Spines	Extremities		Fluoroscopic	Other
			Upper	Lower		
Chest	Skull	Cervical	Hand/finger	Foot/toe	Upper GI/esoph.	
Abdomen	Sinus/facial	Thoracic	Wrist	Ankle	Small bowel	
IVP	Mandible	Lumbar	Forearm	Tibia/fibula	AC BE	
	Orbits/other	Sacrum/coccyx	Elbow	Knee	BE	
			Humerus	Femur		
			Shoulder	Hip		
			Clavicle/scapula	Pelvis		

Complete the columns below by filling in the total number of views for each category of procedures taken for each date.

Torso	Head	Spine	Extremity	Fluoroscopic	Other

TOTAL FOR PERIOD—Add each column   **GRAND TOTAL**

Total number of views for the period (add all columns):   _____

Radiation Protection: Distance Versus Shielding

Name: _____   Date: _____

The three principle factors of radiation protection are time, distance, and shielding:
Reduce time spent in the vicinity of radiation
Increase the distance from the radiation source
Wear appropriate shielding to attenuate radiation

This lab allows students to compare the reduction in exposure when distance and shielding are used.

Objectives:

Upon completion of this lab, the student will be able to:

1. Demonstrate the proper use of an ionization chamber (R-meter).
2. Compare exposures taken directly in the beam and outside the beam.
3. Compare exposures taken with and without a lead apron.
4. Determine the best combination of factors to achieve the lowest exposure to the technologist.

Materials:

1. Energized x-ray unit
2. Ionization chamber (R-meter)

Procedure:

1. Select a technique that would adequately expose a lateral L-spine. Consult with your instructor as needed.

   _____ kVp   _____ mAs   40 in SID

   1. Place the R-meter directly in the x-ray beam, just outside the beam, and 1 m outside the beam. Record each reading in Data Table as indicated.

2. Repeat the Exposure no. 1, but cover the R-meter with a lead apron for each exposure. Record the reading in Data Table.

3. Answer the analysis questions.

Data:

Exposure No.	Exposure (mR)	% of Exposure No. 1	Exposure with lead apron (mR)	% of Exposure No. 1
1—Directly in the x-ray beam		100%		
2—Just outside the beam				
3—One meter outside the beam				
4—Directly in beam, shielded with lead				

Analysis:

1. Calculate the percentage of dose received for Exposures 2 to 4 by dividing each exposure's mR value by Exposure no. 1's mR value. Multiply your answer times 100 and place your answers in the second column (e.g., Exposure no. 2 mR/Exposure no. 1 mR × 100 = %)

_____

_____

_____

2. Using the exposure values and the % values, place the exposures in order from 1 to 4 with 1 being the highest exposure and 4 the lowest exposure. Evaluate Exposures 2 through 4 to answer a and b.

   a. Which exposure conditions provided the most radiation protection (i.e., least dose)?

_____

_____

b. Which exposure conditions provided the least radiation protection (i.e., most dose)?

_____

_____

3. Based on your answers to Question no. 2, which radiographic principle is the most effective radiation protection measure when used alone: distance or shielding?

_____

_____

_____

4. How can this information be used to lower technologist dose? List at least two guidelines that a technologist should follow in actual practice regarding distance and shielding based on your lab findings.

_____

_____

_____